THE LOGIC OF MADNESS

Also by Matthew Blakeway

The Logic of Self-Destruction

THE LOGIC OF MADNESS

A New Theory of Mental Illness

MATTHEW BLAKEWAY

MEYER LEBOEUF

First published 2016
Meyer LeBoeuf Limited
Genesis 5, Church Lane, Heslington, YORK YO10 5DQ

ISBN 978-0-9927961-3-6 Hardback
ISBN 978-0-9927961-5-0 Paperback
ISBN 978-0-9927961-4-3 ebook
Copyright © Matthew Blakeway 2016

A BIC catalogue record for this book is available from the British Library.

Text design by Georgie Widdrington
Typeset by Ellipsis Digital Limited, Glasgow

Caitlin Johnston
EPG.

CONTENTS

PREFACE

B efore Charles Darwin, a biologist was a chap with a beard and a top hat who tramped through the jungles of Africa. He collected specimens and stuffed them to take home. If he collected anything that nobody with a top hat had seen before, he claimed to have 'discovered' it and gave it a Latin name. When he had collected enough specimens, he could classify them into families, genera and orders—all with Latin names. Darwin's impact was so colossal that it seems reasonable to suggest that biology did not really exist beforehand. It is quite laughable that the mere collection of the racks of specimens that still exist in the basements of our natural history museums was once considered to be science.

Today, a psychiatrist is a physician who tramps through the jungle of a major hospital. They collect specimens of human self-destruction and give them Latin names. When they have enough names, they classify them into groups. Giving names to phenomena for which no explanation exists is no more scientific than it would be if I classified a night-time squeaky floorboard as a 'ghost'. It is quite surprising that psychiatrists do not have top hats, although beards are still in vogue. Many psychiatrists are aware of the scientific limitations in what they do. I met a former psychiatrist who became a general medical practitioner. When I asked him why, he told me that he could diagnose most of his psychiatric patients in five minutes, but then would spend the rest of the session knowing he could do nothing to help them.

Reading various historical surveys of madness, it is astounding how little has changed in our understanding of mental illness. We regularly change names to make them sound more scientific or to appear as medical diagnoses, and this disguises the fact that we still really do not understand how they work. For example, we have stopped calling it 'shell shock' and now call it post-traumatic stress disorder, but there is still little idea of the structure of this condition. We no longer talk of 'maladies of the spirit', but happily distinguish between obsessive-compulsive disorder and obsessive-compulsive personality disorder, and still there is no consensus as to what is going on underneath.

We have replaced terms such as 'insanity' or 'madness' with 'mental illness' because this sounded less derogatory and more medical. But, when it became clear that we could not demonstrate something wrong with the physical or chemical working of the body or brain, we started to doubt that these were true medical illnesses; so now we prefer to term them as 'mental disorders'. This, of course, presumes that the word 'mental' has a clear agreed meaning. But if you read the philosophical literature on problems of mind or free will, you will notice that it certainly does not. It also presumes that such conditions are disordered and, as I hope to show, they actually have a definable order. In past centuries, the bourgeoisie would go to mental hospitals (that were really prisons) to look at the insane as a sort of respectable amusement. These days, we would consider such voyeurism to be abhorrent, but the prejudice surrounding mental illness has hardly abated and we prefer these things to be swept out of sight—so has this really changed?

In America, the bible of psychiatry is called the *Diagnostic and Statistical Manual of Mental Disorders, Fifth Edition* (which I refer to as DSM-V and for earlier editions I refer to DSM-IV, DSM-III or DSM-II as applicable, or I refer to them collectively as DSM). The title is perhaps a giveaway, but this book does little more than describe symptoms, classify them together in correlated groups and give them names. Outside America, the standard reference is the *International Statistical Classification of Diseases and Related Health Problems, 10th Revision* (which I refer to as ICD-10), produced by the World Health Organization. Throughout this book, I will refer mostly to DSM. In sciences like physics and biology where the extent of our knowledge is vast, scientists tend to be open and honest about what they do not understand. By contrast, in psychiatry we understand very little about the mechanisms of the conditions that scientists observe. This relative lack of knowledge makes specialists in the field a little defensive. It is one of the universal rules of science that if you are unable to explain something, you give it a Latin name, so that you can sound erudite even when selectively ignorant. You are now deemed an 'expert', and you get to write the speculative obfuscatory description of its causes sprinkled with words like 'epiphenomenal'.

The aim of this book is to create a hypothetical theoretical framework of what mental illness actually is. In *The Logic of Self-Destruction*,[1] I explained that self-destructive actions are rationally derived. To do this, I described an algorithm of how a human computes an action. The transition from ordinary human self-destruction to mental illness requires us to develop these ideas to a higher level of complexity. Mental illness is self-destruction taken to the next dimension. When a cue ball strikes a billiard ball, it flies off in a predictable direction. If the billiard ball is simultaneously struck by two cue balls, the two causes combine to produce one effect and mechanics permits us to predict in which direction the billiard ball will travel. If a self-destructive action is the rational consequence of manipulated emotional behaviour that started out as a tactical deception, what happens if behaviour is manipulated in two different ways simultaneously? This combination should not cause two self-destructive actions, but a single one, and it is a safe bet that it will be more seriously self-destructive. To work out what this looks like, we have to consider how the two causes combine, and compute the effect. In this way, we can predict self-destructive actions of a higher degree of complexity.

Even psychiatrists sometimes describe their patients as being irrational, but the concept of 'irrationality' is scientifically so incoherent that it is not even wrong. My aim is to demonstrate that all the symptoms described in the DSM can be derived logically. Even the mad are rational. I may not complete my intended task, but even getting halfway could reorient how we understand mental illness and this step could be the beginning of psychiatry as a scientific discipline with an explanatory causal theory.

I am attacking the idea of mental illness and placing patterns of extreme self-destructiveness into a broad spectrum of what makes us human. Having obsessive-compulsive disorder, being a member of the Tea Party, being a Hindu, and being in love with someone who abuses you are *all* obsessive-compulsive. Comparisons between religious belief, radical ideology and mental illness have been frequently made (for example, by Sam Harris[2]). Nothing gives a psychiatrist the right to call any one of these a 'disorder' (except of course their self-granted right), and nothing gives Richard Dawkins the right to hold religious people up for ridicule. As far back as the nineteenth century, doctors included being too religious as a category of mental illness, so today they could also include being politically left wing, and the psychiatric profession in China could include being right wing.

The thesis of this book is that madness is logical in structure; not 'psycho'- or 'neuro'-logical, but plain old-skool logical. This is the way that Aristotle would understand it—one of the earliest thinkers from ancient Greece to set out a formal description of logic. Psychiatry, like pre-Darwinian biology, is pre-scientific in that it describes phenomena without having any convincing, explanatory theory. This book provides an explanatory theory, but a surprising conclusion of this book is how much psychiatry got right without any theory of causality. That is because being *pre*-scientific does not mean being *un*scientific. Many scientists working in a field before it had any causal theory were performing research of high scientific diligence. Consider Galileo, who, by telescopic observation, provided evidence for the Copernican theory that the Earth orbited the Sun rather than the other way round—despite not being able to explain why. Also, Darwin's work before he came up with his theory of natural selection—the fundamental causal theory of biology—was scrupulously well observed and documented. Most scientists researching mental disorders are following diligent scientific practice in a pre-scientific field. This book supports most of the distinctions they have made. For example, acute personality disorder remains as a distinct category, not because it has distinct symptoms, but because it has a distinct structure. And the distinction between the spectra of human self-destruction that psychiatrists used to call 'neurosis' and 'psychosis' largely remains intact—maybe with the boundaries slightly shifted. Psychiatry has been accused of being pseudoscientific or unscientific, but this is completely unfair and its critics have generally not been too scientific themselves. Being unscientific refers to bad practice, but you can follow good pre-scientific practice if you enquire diligently in the absence of a causal theory. However, the pre-scientific nature of psychiatry occasionally makes it prone to losing its way, not only scientifically, but also morally. This is generally recognised within psychiatry. Two respected psychiatrists, Richard Hunter and Ida Macalpine, summed it up like this:

> There is not even an objective method of describing or communicating clinical findings without subjective interpretations and no exact uniform terminology which conveys precisely the same to all. In consequence there is wide divergence of diagnosis, even of diagnoses, a steady flow of new terms and an ever-changing nomenclature, as well as a surfeit of hypotheses which tend to be presented as fact. Furthermore, aetiology remains speculative, pathogenesis largely obscure, classifications predominantly symptomatic and hence arbitrary and possibly ephemeral; physical treatments are empirical and subject to fashion, and psychotherapies still only in their infancy and doctrinaire.[3]

Psychiatry's pre-scientific nature leads me to reject its jargon—rather like a modern biologist who has little time for all the Latin names of the species. Since it is mostly concerned with describing symptoms, psychiatry has a rich jargon for effects, but little for causes. When I describe a generic causal structure for an 'Anti-

Compulsion', I am actually not that concerned with what the effect is. Someone can have an Anti-Compulsion with respect to eating (for which a psychiatrist uses the Latin name 'anorexia nervosa') or talking (which is described as 'mutism'), but to me there is little difference between them. Once you have a causal theory for these conditions, it makes little sense to group together Anti-Compulsions with respect to eating with other 'eating disorders' when they clearly have separate causal mechanisms. This is like grouping lung cancer and the common cold as 'breathing disorders', which of course we probably would group if we had no idea of the causes or mechanisms of such diseases.

It might seem callous of me to totally disregard the patient, but this cuts both ways. I cannot judge a compulsive serial killer because judgement gets in the way of analysis of the cause; so too does compassion for someone who has a compulsion to wash their hands. Suspension of both judgement and compassion dispels the confusion that morality places on this understanding. It is ridiculous that we should think of a compulsive serial killer as *evil* and someone with another compulsion as being pitiable, since neither of them has a choice about where their compulsion leads. We judge the former morally because they harm others, whereas the latter only harms them, but this is not a choice for either. Everybody has self-destructive urges, and we are merely fortunate if we have fewer urges than others, or ones that are easier to contain or which are morally acceptable in the society in which we happen to live.

Matthew Blakeway, 2016

A:
FOUNDATIONS

One day perhaps, we will no longer
know what madness was.
— Michel Foucault, History of Madness

THE CONCEPT OF MADNESS

THE HISTORY OF WHAT WE HAVE CALLED IT

Madness, melancholy, insanity, lunacy, craziness, unsound mind, mental disorder, unreason, loco, mental illness—a dizzying array of words has been used to describe a condition that we have never truly understood. In each age, there has been an accepted way of discussing this subject depending upon how the condition was perceived. The term 'lunacy', for example, stems from the ancient belief that madness was caused by the moon. The classical term was 'melancholy', even though it was recognised this could include unreasonable ecstasy. In times when madness was seen as benign, people with this condition were known as 'holy fools' or 'idiots'. In times when madness was feared or subject to prejudice, the terms used sounded derogatory, such as 'insanity' or 'unreason'. When philanthropists, such as Daniel Tuke, took over responsibility for the management of the mad in the eighteenth century, we changed the terms to reflect a more humane approach. He adopted the French term 'mental alienation'. This, he said 'conveys a more just idea of this disorder, than those expressed which imply, in any degree, the "abolition of the thinking capacity"'.[4] Then, in the nineteenth century, physicians became involved in the study of madness, and we started to call it 'mental illness'. General concept words started to sound technical, medical, or were simply spoken in Latin.

Sigmund Freud completely changed how we talked about and understood ourselves, where everything was discussed in terms of madness. For half a century after his death, everybody thought that he or she was a psychiatrist, and it was normal to diagnose your own neuroses and complexes, as well as those of your friends. Everybody was a 'crazy mixed-up kid'. These ideas were applied to society as a whole, ultimately leading to the 'psychiatrisation' of everything. Even sociology became a branch of psychiatry with widespread talk of juvenile delinquency and the degenerate society.

Psychiatry today tends to avoid the term 'mental illness', since an illness implies something wrong with the functioning of the physical body. Instead, the term 'mental disorder' is considered more appropriate. This change of nomenclature does not disguise the fact that the field of psychiatry is still not certain whether mental disorders are caused by a malfunction with the physical brain, such as a neurological or chemical cause, or something 'psychological'.

To date, there has been no agreed causal theory of madness. We do not even have an explanation of what madness is. We just think we know what it looks like. This is little different from the situation that existed in the seventeenth century. Changing the terms we use disguises the fact that psychiatry is still not even a *young* science. It cannot become a science until it has consensus regarding a structural theory.

The general aim of my work is to put psychology on the same shelf as alchemy. I do not understand what psychology is or what it is trying to prove. This book will not give madness a new name, but it will explain a theory on how it works and create some new technical terms for different structures. These structures are logical in nature, and once we realise this, perhaps we will need to change the way we talk about madness yet again.

THE HISTORY OF CLASSIFICATION

In the absence of any causal theory, all we can do is set out classificatory systems. This is a branch of medicine known as nosology, and a nosologist is a person who classifies diseases. The approach of the Diagnostic and Statistical Manual (DSM) is essentially nosological. But to put where we are now into context, we need to look at the history of the concept and classification of madness from the earliest times until the present day. In some ways, it has not changed that much but, as I will explore, there are a finite number of logical structures for madness, and scientists and doctors through the ages have been able to spot their different characteristics without understanding the underlying mechanisms.

Michel Foucault examined madness from a historical and philosophical perspective in his landmark book *The History of Madness*.[5] This covers the evolving concept of madness from medieval times until just prior to Freud at the beginning of the twentieth century. At the beginning of this period, madness was considered to be a form of punishment sent by God, and it was evidence of moral failings. Doctors and scientists today regard this notion as severely outdated, but our concepts of madness and criminality remain utterly confused, and occasionally interchangeable. I will explore this more fully in one of the closing chapters in this book: The Poor, the Mad and the Criminal. The first attempts to classify mental disorders in a scientific fashion emerged in the late Renaissance. One of the first to put together a system was Paracelsus, a sixteenth-century scientist and polymath. His classification of the various forms of madness was as follows:

> The '*Lunatici*', whose sickness had the moon at its origin, and whose behaviour, in its apparent irregularity, was secretly ordered by its phases and movements. The '*Insani*' owed their condition to heredity, unless they had contracted it, just before their birth, in their mother's womb; the '*Vesani*' were deprived of reason and sense through the abuse of alcohol or through bad food, and the '*Melancholici*' were inclined towards madness by some vice in their nature.[6]

From the beginning of the seventeenth century, these classifications started to become more detailed. Huge work was put into these schemes, but they were all rapidly abandoned because none had any theoretical hypothesis beyond mere classification. The frequency of new schemes was almost equivalent to the rate at which the committee of the DSM puts out new editions, but these earlier schemes generally had no institutional backing because there was no professional body coordinating efforts. However, some of the psychiatric

classifications that we recognise today have precedents that date back
a surprisingly long time. In fact, the diagnoses of mental diseases are
often older than the diagnoses of physical ones. For example:

- Hysteria is perhaps the oldest recognised mental disorder and
  was first described by ancient Egyptian physicians. The name
  is derived from the ancient Greek word for the womb and it
  was supposed that the condition resulted from displacement
  of the womb. Hysteria is no longer officially a recognised
  condition, but a similar institutional medical sexism still
  lingers with histrionic personality disorder.

- The modern concept of bipolar disorder was included in
  most historical classifications by its original name of
  'melancholia' as far back as Hippocrates in 400 BC. Robert
  Burton described hypomania in the early seventeenth century
  as: 'humorous they are beyond all measure, sometimes
  profusely laughing, extraordinarily merry, and then again
  weeping without a cause';[7] and the English doctor Thomas
  Willis set out a more scientific description using the term
  'manic depression' later that century.[8]

- The Scottish doctor William Cullen was probably the first to
  use the term 'neurosis' in 1769, and Karl Friedrich Canstatt
  coined the term 'psychosis' (an abbreviation of 'psychic
  neurosis') in 1841. Scientists and doctors were generally
  agreed upon the distinction between neurosis and psychosis
  by the middle of the nineteenth century. The latter appears to
  involve a complete loss of touch with reality. In recent times,
  there is a tendency to stop using the term 'neurosis'.

- Weickhard was one of the earliest doctors to describe
  'attention deficit'. He mentioned it in 1790 in his *Der
  Philosophische Arzt*.[9]

- The symptoms of schizophrenia were described in antiquity,
  for example, by Hippocrates: 'In some cases the girl says
  dreadful things: [the visions] order her to jump up and throw
  herself into wells and drown, as if this were good for her and

served some useful purpose';[10] and also by Aretaeus in the first century AD: 'One believes himself a sparrow; or cock or an earthen vase; one believes himself a God, orator or actor, carrying gravely a stalk of straw and imagining himself holding a sceptre of the world; some utter cries of an infant and demand to be carried in arms, or they believe themselves a grain of mustard, and tremble continuously for fear of being eaten by a hen.'[11] In 1809, the French physician Philippe Pinel described it more scientifically, although he used its classical Latin name of *dementia praecox*. Emil Kraepelin further refined his description at the end of the nineteenth century, although it was not until the twentieth century that Kurt Schneider defined a more scientific separation of schizophrenia from other syndromes.

- The recognition of personality disorder probably also started with Pinel, who recognised '*manie sans délire*', or 'mania without delirium'.[12] This was a new observation because previously, delusion was considered to be a central component of psychiatric disorders.

By the eighteenth century, most classificatory systems were already starting to resemble simplified versions of the DSM. One example, given by Foucault, was authored by Linnaeus in 1763[13] as follows:

Class V: Mental Maladies:
1. Ideal: delirium, transport, dementia, mania, demonomania and melancholy.
2. Imaginative: tinnitus, visions, vertigo, panicky terror, hypochondria and somnambulism.
3. Pathetic: depraved tastes, bulimia, polydipsia, satyriasis, erotomania, nostalgia, Saint Vitus dance, rage, hydrophobia, cacosity, antipathy and anxiety.

Early classifications nearly always included hypochondria. But around 1725, hypochondria and hysteria increasingly merged into one condition, since imagining you were ill was seen as an hysterical symptom.[14] However, this is little different to the DSM of today, where new categories appear and others merge with each new edition. Looking at broader categorisations, the term 'neurosis' is now officially dropped from the lexicon, so too in its turn was 'hysteria'. Homosexuality and masturbation have all disappeared from official psychiatric manuals and are now recognised as normal behaviours. More recently, 'Asperger's syndrome' was eliminated in DSM–5, becoming merged into the autism spectrum.

However, some very old behaviour patterns are making a new appearance after ages of obscurity. 'Social anxiety disorder' (previously known as 'shyness') did not appear until DSM–III, despite the fact that Hippocrates described it fairly accurately two and a half millennia ago:

> Through bashfulness, suspicion, and timorousness, will not be seen abroad, loves darkness as life and cannot endure the light or to sit in lightsome places, his hat still in his eyes, he will neither see nor be seen by his good will. He dare not come in company for fear he should be misused, disgraced, overshoot himself in gesture or speeches, or be sick; he thinks every man observes him, aims at him, derides him, owes him malice.[15]

These comings and goings of classification have been occurring since the dawn of science, but none of this is actually scientifically justifiable. People who called themselves scientists merely created a classification and as Thomas Szasz, a Hungarian-American psychiatrist claimed, 'Freud did not *discover* that hysteria was a mental illness. He merely asserted and advocated that so-called hysterics be *declared* ill.'[16] Each generation of doctors is committed to their own classification, but the constant changing, with disappointingly little emergence of a consensus theory of causality, should eliminate confidence in any informed observer.

THE HISTORY OF THE THEORIES OF CAUSES

Theories of the causes of madness first started to appear in ancient Greece. Plato's view is an example of such early ideas:

> We must allow that disease of the soul is senselessness; and of this there are two forms, madness and stupidity. Every condition then in which a man suffers from either of these must be termed a disease. We must also affirm that the gravest maladies of the soul are excessive pleasures or pains. For if a man is under the influence of excessive joy, or on the other hand, of extreme pain, and is eager unduly to grasp the one or shun the other, he is able neither to see nor to hear anything aright; he is delirious, and at that moment entirely unable to obey reason.[17]

Hippocrates, as previously quoted, also made many observations of psychiatric conditions and described them in ways that are recognisable today, but he offered little by way of explanations. Aristotle and Pliny the Elder[18] were early proponents of the idea that 'lunacy' was caused by the phases of the moon. Astonishingly, this latter theory is not dead, and a casual internet search will turn up a number of recent articles, some of them in respectable journals.

Burton's *The Anatomy of Melancholy*, written in 1621, lists so many causes that it is a wonder that anybody was normal. 'He that begets a child on a full stomach will either have a sick child or a crazed son.'[19] However, he saw the causes as broadly falling into three categories:

> The first proceeds from the sole fault of the brain, and is called head-melancholy; the second sympathetically proceeds from the whole body, when the whole temperature is melancholy: the third ariseth from the bowels, liver, spleen, or membrane called mesenterium, named hypochondriacal or windy melancholy . . .[20]

Adopting a morality of moderation in all things, Burton frequently lists too much of something being a cause, and then too little of the same being a cause of another form of 'melancholy'. For example: 'If the brain be hot, the animal spirits are hot; much madness follows, with violent actions: if cold, fatuity and sottishness'.[21] The cause of melancholy to which he devotes most attention is 'love of learning, or overmuch study',[22] which is ironic given that, comprising over half a million words and referencing hundreds of sources, his vast book was clearly not under-researched. Perhaps Burton needed to create such a large body of work because he thought the symptoms of melancholia within the mind were infinite.[23] He was, however, convinced that the causes were not mystical:

> A better means in my judgement cannot be taken than to show them the causes whence they proceed; not from devils as they suppose, or that they are bewitched or forsaken of God, hear or see, etc., as many of them think, but from natural and inward causes; that so knowing them, they may better avoid the effects, or at least endure them with more patience. The most grievous and common symptoms are fear and sorrow, and that without a cause to the wisest and discreetest men, in this malady not to be avoided.[24]

Throughout the Age of Enlightenment, the concept of madness was dominated by the distinction between reason and unreason. For example, the definition of madness in the *Encyclopédie* from the first half of the eighteenth century was as follows:

> To stray unwittingly from the path of reason because one has no ideas, is to be an imbecile; knowingly to stray from the path when one is prey to a violent passion is to be weak; but to walk confidently away from it, with the firm persuasion that one is following it, that, it seems to me, is what is genuinely called mad.[25]

As Foucault points out, this concept of reason and unreason creates a paradox: the contradiction of believing one is following the path of reason when one is not makes it logically impossible for a madman to know he is mad. Only one who is sane can tell when someone is mad. Unreason stands in opposition to reason, whose only content is reason itself. Therefore, when somebody says 'that man is mad' this statement is not based on any theory of what madness actually is.

The gradual abandonment of the idea of unreason, combined with the development of more humane ways of managing the mad, prompted the philosopher Georg Hegel to pronounce:

> The right psychical treatment therefore keeps in view the truth that insanity is not an abstract loss of reason (neither in the point of intelligence nor of will and its responsibility), but only derangement, only a contradiction in a still subsisting reason;—just as physical disease is not an abstract, i.e. mere and total, loss of health (if it were that, it would be death), but a contradiction in it. This humane treatment, no less benevolent than reasonable (the services of Pinel towards which deserve the highest acknowledgement), presupposes the patient's rationality, and in that assumption has the sound basis for dealing with him on this side—just as in the case of bodily disease the physician bases his treatment on the vitality which as such still contains health.[26]

Hegel is praising the emergence of a more humanitarian perspective on madness. This also involves an abandonment of the idea of unreason and suggests that the cause of madness is actually rational, but Hegel does not offer a theory as to how this actually works. This absence of a causal theory has been the undoing of psychiatry as a scientific project.

The discoveries that certain forms of madness had origins in organic medical conditions proved to be a red herring that was hard to escape. For example, in 1838, Jean-Étienne Dominique Esquirol demonstrated that epilepsy is an organic disease. And in 1858, Guillaume Duchenne demonstrated that a loss of ability to coordinate movement, known as *tabes dorsalis,* was caused by syphilis. Initially, these discoveries gave scientists optimism that we would soon work out the causes of all madness, but this confidence was short-lived. What happened instead was that such conditions were reclassified from psychiatry to neurology or some other branch of medicine. And the madness that was left remained without an explanation.

Throughout history, many scientists have posited the causes of madness with unshakeable certainty. Early physicians and scientists spent much time dissecting the brains of mad people to discover what was wrong with them. Each of them had a theory: the brains of hysterics were too waxy, less dense, or wetter, and the brains of melancholics were less flexible, denser, drier, etc. The scientific confidence of the Age of Enlightenment led scientists to believe that all madness was classifiable and its causes analysable, but the explanations given at the time seem to be beyond anything that we would call science today. Some of these hypothesised causes, in hindsight, were almost as mad as what they were trying to explain. For example, in the seventeenth century it was assumed that madness was caused by a 'morbiffick matter'[27] and, although there was no recognisably scientific explanation of what this was, there was much debate as to how one could detect its presence.

One example of a doctor having unjustified confidence in the power of his own knowledge was William Black, who analysed the mad in Bethlem Hospital in London between 1772 and 1787. He described their causes:

> A hereditary disposition, drunkenness, excessive study, fevers, the consequences of childbirth, obstructions of the viscera, bruises and fractures, venereal disease, small pox, ulcers that dry too quickly, upsets, worries and misfortunes, love, jealousy, excessive devotion or belonging to a Methodist sect, pride.[28]

The penultimate one is my favourite! Another physician who was overly confident of his knowledge of causes was the Frenchman Giraudy, who determined the causes of mental illness in patients at Charenton mental hospital in 1804:

One hundred and fifty are ill as a result of powerful afflictions of the soul, such as jealousy, disappointment in love, excessive joy, ambition, fear, terror or intense sadness; 52 have inherited their condition; for 28 it is a result of masturbation; 3, a syphilitic virus; 12, the abuse of the pleasures of Venus; 31, the abuse of alcoholic beverages; 12, the abuse of their intellectual faculties; for 2 it is the result of worms in the intestine; one the consequences of scabies; for 5 it is the result of herpes; 29, of milky metastasis; and 2, sunstroke.[29]

The idea that the cause of madness was a moral fault survived until the end of the nineteenth century.

Hysteria was long considered to be exclusive to women. Prior to the eighteenth century, it was thought to be the result of a displacement of the womb. By the mid-eighteenth century, some considered hysteria to be caused by the fermentation of salts after they came into contact with alkaline; while others thought it was caused by yeast coming into contact with too much acidity.[30]

To add to the array of possible causes, we then have to consider the distinction between neurological and psychological causes. In the late nineteenth century, Wilhelm Greisinger claimed that 'psychological diseases are diseases of the brain. Insanity itself ... is only a symptom.'[31] This was a brave statement of what was widely accepted in Germany in the nineteenth century, but nobody was able to produce scientific evidence of it. This line of reasoning assumed that all madness was a product of a damaged brain, and buried the idea of psychological causes. Greisinger argued for the merging of psychiatry and neurology, ignoring psychology. Karl Wernicke continued this work in Germany. He became interested in 'aphasia' (a loss of ability to understand or express speech) and how it correlated with brain damage. Of course, some mental illnesses were discovered to have a physical cause in the brain, such as epilepsy, beriberi or neurosyphilis. But the discovery of the cause results in these illnesses ceasing to be a form of psychopathology and they are reclassified as a form of neuropathology. That is fine, except that we do not know what psychopathology really is.

The shift from neurological causes to psychological causes started with Jean-Martin Charcot (1825–1893), a neurologist and neuropathologist working in Paris. Charcot was a nosographer—he merely classified diseases. However, since in his day all neurological conditions were incurable, his interest shifted from neurological diseases to conditions that merely imitated them. He started on the path that led to the differentiation between neurology and psychiatry. Before Charcot, a person was ill if something was wrong with his body of a physico-chemical nature, and people who pretended that something was wrong were malingerers. The physician had to be able to determine the difference between real and imaginary illnesses—the sick and the malingerer. And since malingerers were trying to deceive the physician, they earned the physician's scorn.

An hysteric is someone who experiences some form of unmanageable emotional excess. Charcot threw his considerable reputation and scientific knowledge behind the fact that hysterics were not malingerers. But he never produced any solid evidence for this, and his case was significantly undermined by the later discovery that his assistants kept Charcot happy by schooling patients at Salpêtrière to imitate the symptoms of hysteria.[32] This is a confusing situation for any doctor or scientist to confront, since the people he or she is observing might be imitating the imitation of sickness. Where does one begin?

Freud, who was Charcot's student, completed the shift from a neurological approach to one that was entirely psychological. A malingerer could impersonate a neurological disease, and this became known as hysteria. But the symptoms of hysteria could be impersonated too. Freud effectively solved this problem, by declaring that malingering was an illness too. The unconscious impersonation of illness is an illness, whereas the conscious impersonation of illness is malingering. It would appear that only Freud and his followers are qualified to tell whether an illness without a physical cause has a conscious or unconscious origin.

In 1916, Freud started with the theory that hysteria in women was the result of prepubescent seduction, often by the father. His colleague Josef Breuer continued with this theory, but Freud abandoned it, replacing it with the idea of the 'Oedipus Complex': children are in love with their opposite sex parent but jealous of their same sex parent. Later, this expanded into ideas of the 'id, ego and superego', together with the 'death instinct'. He then went on to develop his ideas of the unconscious mind and how difficult memories and experiences were repressed. These, he claimed, resurfaced to cause neurotic symptoms. Towards the end of his life, he expanded his theories to cover the origins of incest taboos, monotheism, and the whole gamut of anthropological and cultural phenomena.

Carl Jung took Freud's ideas to even greater extremes. He collaborated with Freud from 1907 to 1912, when they abruptly split. Jung took the idea of the unconscious mind and elevated it to a social phenomenon: the collective unconscious. But, by this stage, he appeared to have lost all pretence of being scientific and was unapologetic about his mysticism and pseudo-religion. Jung reduced madness to the mystical, with talk about the collective unconscious of distant ancestral memories and myths of the Earth Mother. Karl Popper lambasted all of these ideas as being pseudoscientific, because they had the character of myths and could not be tested by experimental method. He claimed that 'science must begin with myths, and with the criticism of myths.'[33] Freud and Jung thought that religion was a form of madness that was discoverable by psychoanalysis, but neither of them realised that they had invented a religion of their own.

Despite the doubts about the scientific credentials of Charcot, Freud, Jung and their followers, these ideas survived well into the twentieth century. Kurt Eissler, a Viennese-American psychiatrist working at the time of World War II, declared:

It can be rightly claimed that malingering is always the sign of a disease often more severe than a neurotic disorder because it

concerns an arrest of development at an early phase. It is a disease
which to diagnose requires particularly keen diagnostic acumen.
The diagnosis should never be made but by the psychiatrist. It is a
great mistake to make a patient suffering from the disease liable to
prosecution, at least if he falls within the type of personality I have
described here.[34]

R. D. Laing considered himself a Freudian, yet he developed a theory
of schizophrenia that did not draw upon supposed causes in the
unconscious. He claimed that a normal 'embodied' person has a sense
of identity that is at one with his body or mind. The person sees his
perceptions of the outside world as real and his actions as purposeful.
When a person sees his actions as futile—for example, because his
parents ignored him—then he comes to despise or fear his real self,
and develops a fantasy self that brings greater fulfilment than the real
one. This false-self starts to disembody and the sense of self trans-
forms:

Instead of: (self/body) ←→ other
We have: self ←→ (body-other).[35]

Over time this leads to a split between a true (unsatisfactory) self
and a cultivated false-self system. 'Objects of fantasy or imagination
obey magical laws; they have magical relationships, not real relationships.'[36] Gradually the false-self system becomes more extensive
and then more autonomous. It starts to become 'harassed' by compulsive behaviour fragments. Eventually, all that belongs to it
becomes more and more dead, unreal, false and mechanical.

Laing became hugely influential in British psychiatry and became
a cult-bestseller, in part because of the way he wrote about alienation in the era of the Vietnam War and Pink Floyd's *Dark Side of
the Moon*. But gradually, even these views faded, because like most
theories in psychiatry, they relied upon the type of explanation that
diligent scientists and mathematicians pejoratively call 'hand-waving'

explanations. Their vagueness meant that they could not be put to empirical test.

Today, the theories of the causes of 'mental disorders' have yet to completely throw off the pseudoscientific theories of Freud and show little narrowing of consensus. The intellectual descendants of Freud propound theories based in relationships with mothers, concepts of the self, developmental frameworks, etc. But when we survey the spectrum, we can find neither a robust neurological theory, nor a psychological one. As scepticism with Freud grows, the pendulum is swinging back towards mental disorders having biological causes within the brain. Much research is devoted to performing brain scans on people with such disorders in the hope that we might stumble upon a new clue. Often, when such clues are found, it is difficult to know what they mean. For example, people with depression have low levels of serotonin in their brains, but it is difficult to know how this fits into the causal structure of the condition. Even if such research does not lead to a convergence upon a consensus theory, at least it *feels* like 'proper' science, and that is the best we can hope for at the moment.

THE HISTORY OF 'CURES'

If the historic explanations of madness were often themselves mad, some of the historic ideas of cures were even worse. Opium was often used as a 'cure', and doctors prescribed all sorts of human tissues as medicine. Human hair was burnt and inhaled—this was considered as a cure for the 'vapours'. The prize for the most bizarre 'cure' was the ground skull of a hanged man, which some recommended as a cure for convulsions, spasms and epilepsy.[37] Francis Willis, a British doctor who achieved fame by treating one of the most famous madmen of all, King George III, would fix his patients with a piercing stare—a mesmeric technique for gaining mastery over them.

From the seventeenth century onwards there was generally little hope of curing madness. The usual response was mass incarceration of the mad in prison-like asylums, with conditions so abominable that they became a subject of fascination. Raving patients were chained to beds, straightjacketed and generally treated worse than animals. This approach changed with the broader shift in ideas that came with the Age of Enlightenment in the late eighteenth century. From the Enlightenment perspective, knowledge and science should serve human objectives, rather than supposed divine ones. Madness was no longer seen as a punishment sent by God. Therefore, those caring for mad people are obligated to do so in a humane way.

Pinel insisted that the insane in the hospitals that he managed, Bicêtre and Salpêtrière, should be unchained. He was usually seen as liberating the mad, but he held that they should be treated by 'moral methods' and, in many ways, this was just a different form of control. Samuel Tuke, a Quaker from a family of mental health reformers, employed similar methods in England. He believed in religious segregation and the moral teaching that this entailed—in effect, he adopted a praying cure.

Pinel, by contrast, noted that a great many of his patients were Catholics, and considered 'religious madness' to be a recognisable condition. Pinel himself was a Catholic and had previously considered becoming a priest. He preferred religion was kept out of his treatment, but remained convinced that married women were less likely to suffer from hysteria than young girls, and that many conditions were caused by excessive drunkenness and extreme promiscuity. Pinel's asylums became places of moral uniformity and instruction, and madness was seen as a form of degeneration. Punishments, including ice-cold showers, were meted out for minor infractions such as not eating one's food. And although the patients were free to wander unchained and unconstrained, they were threatened with restraint if they did not comply, and were frequently humiliated for their madness.

Medicine became a form of justice and therapeutics turned into repression. This was an imprisonment in a moral world where freedom could only be won by repentance. Tuke and Pinel might have been reformers of different philosophies, but there was one thing they agreed on: the shift from confinement of the insane to their care in humane hospitals meant that doctors should supervise them. This gave rise to the modern notion of mental illness being an illness, rather than madness being an affliction. Still, our understanding of mental illness remained pre-scientific, and the role of the doctor as healer was not scientific but almost mystical.

Even in the eighteenth century, doctors recognised that their cures for madness were not scientific. Physicians themselves did not hand out medicines; rather these came from empirics. This division of responsibilities meant that neither party was responsible for cures that did not work (i.e. all of them).[38]

By 1900, all confidence that insanity could be cured had vanished. Fears grew that insanity might be an epidemic, and ideas of incarceration, eugenics and sterilisation became debated, both in America and Germany. At this time, madness was one of the few criteria for being refused immigration into America. Ellis Island, where most immigration was processed, has a derelict mental hospital round the back. Most of the island is now a beautiful museum, but the United States National Park Service would rather avoid embarrassing questions about the fate of those prospective immigrants who ended up in there. Eugenic policies targeting the mentally ill with sterilisation were quite common throughout the world in the early twentieth century; for example, America, Sweden and Switzerland, all passed laws for mandatory sterilisation of various people, including certain types of mental illness. It was almost inevitable that in the 1930s, the Nazis in Germany would progress from eugenic sterilisation to eugenic euthanasia. Nazi psychiatry determined that the lives of schizophrenics were not 'worth living' and plans were made for their annihilation along with all other victims of the Holocaust. The Germans secretly code-named this, the T4 programme, which was active from 1939 to 1941 and named after its Berlin headquarters at Tiergartenstrasse 4. Such policies seem horrific today, but they partly reflect the level of despair that scientists and doctors had of ever solving the problem. And the scale of the problem was immense: at its peak the population of mental hospitals in America was approximately 0.5 per cent of the entire population of the country.[39]

Freud's theories of neurosis led him to develop psychoanalysis, and this appeared to be the first likely attempt to get to the bottom of the matter in a scientific manner. He abolished the moral condemnation of his predecessors and so released mental illness from its moral cage. But he retained the mystical relationship between doctor and patient that had been introduced by Pinel and Tuke. Prior to Freud, physicians saw themselves as sane people studying the insane, but Freud turned this on its head: we should understand all humanity in terms of insanity, because all of us have some insanity inside. There emerged a tripartite understanding: man, his madness and his truth, which replaced the understanding of the eighteenth century of the binary division of reason and unreason, truth and error, reality and delusion.

Jung and Freud's collaboration gave rise to a whole range of therapies, from hypnosis to free association. They gave talk therapy a respectability that it had previously lacked. Freud's id–ego–super-ego model of the mind gave birth to the drive theory. In America psychoanalysts focused on development functions of the ego, which came to be known as ego psychology, while in Europe psychoanalysts focused on the early mother–infant relationship believed to be most important in the development of psychological traits. Freud himself was highly focused on sexual stimuli as a source of psychological disturbance, but among psychoanalysts today who consider themselves Freudians, the importance of this is greatly diminished. However, the success of their methods was always in doubt, and there were even allegations that Freud doctored his notes to bolster the results that he hoped for. In Britain, where Freud worked at the end of his life, these ideas were met with scepticism. In 1916, Charles Mercier, a British psychiatrist noted:

> Psychoanalysis is past its perihelion, and is rapidly retreating into the dark and silent depths from which it emerged. It is well that it

should be systematically described before it goes to join pounded toads and sour milk in the limbo of discarded remedies.[40]

But the horrors of World War I and the phenomenon of 'shell shock' caused a huge upsurge in British psychiatry. With so many patients coming back from the trenches unable to walk, talk, see or hear, with seemingly no physical cause, the nascent psychiatric discipline had endless raw material with which to experiment. Psychiatrists such as Ernest Jones set about experimenting with hypnosis to tackle these problems.

The first half of the twentieth century saw doctors experimenting with some barbaric remedies, which were in reality no more humane than the mass incarceration of prior centuries. Julius von Wagner-Jauregg demonstrated that deliberately infecting with malaria was an effective cure for general paresis of the insane (at least of the insanity). In 1920, Manfred Sakel pioneered a technique whereby he injected schizophrenics with insulin to induce a coma in which they remained for sustained periods, occasionally with predictable fatal consequences. Some patients were injected as much as 60 times and placed into a coma as many as 50 times despite showing no signs of improvement[41] This technique was used until the 1960s. Other doctors immersed patients in ice-cold baths, or used chemical or electric shocks to induce convulsions that were sometimes so violent that patients broke their bones. Then, there was a proliferation of attempts to cure madness with brain surgery. Prefrontal lobotomies were used to treat a number of neuroses: surgically separating various parts of the brain from one another. To give you an idea of how invasive this procedure was, here is how one writer described it: 'An instrument resembling an ice pick was inserted under the eyelid through the orbital roof and blindly swept left and right.'[42] Such operations caused unacceptable personality changes, such as loss of attention, responsiveness or inhibition. But over 20,000 such operations were performed in America from the 1930s to the 1950s. All of these treatments could be said to be worse than the disease. It remains something of a scandal that the only specialists in psychiatry to earn a Nobel Prize for medicine were responsible for two of its most horrific mistakes: António Egas Moniz who developed lobotomy techniques and the aforementioned von Wagner-Jauregg.[43] However, to put this into context, we need to remember that American psychiatric hospitals contained hundreds of thousands of patients for whom there really was no other hope.

In 1949, psychopharmacology was born. Lithium emerged as an effective treatment to manage bipolar disorder. (At the time, it was called manic depression.) This was the first of a long series of drugs that altered the symptoms of mental disorders. Largactyl came shortly after, and this drug was so notorious that its critics mocked it as the 'liquid cosh' due to its effect of rendering patients almost incapable of doing anything. This movement inspired a new confidence (after centuries of despondency) that symptoms could be alleviated. It also gave psychiatry new pretentions to be a medical science of equal standing to, for example, oncology or haematology. Psychopharmacological drugs might be developed in laboratories, but much science is performed away from laboratories and much of what occurs in laboratories *is not* science. The scientific limitation that overhangs most of these drugs is that we might know *how* they work, but we still have no idea *why* they work, because we have no idea about the causal structure of the symptoms we are treating. We would do well to remember what Galen said in the second century BC, 'It is in vain to speak of cures, or think of remedies, until such time as we have considered of the causes.'[44] If we do not know the cause of a symptom, which in these cases is actually a form of behaviour, then a 'cure' is anything that makes the symptom disappear—simply a change in behaviour. This is a considerable dilution of the concept of a 'cure' as a cancer doctor would understand it. These days, most medical science outside psychiatry has a very good understanding of both why and how drugs work. But the drugs prescribed by psychiatrists are almost purely palliative: they lessen symptoms without understanding the cause of the symptom.

For example, most antipsychotic drugs 'work' by changing the way the brain processes dopamine, but nobody understands how dopamine fits into the causal structure of the psychosis in the first place, so we do not know *why* this works. In a later chapter in this book (Intentional Delusions), I offer a novel hypothesis of the linkage between dopamine and schizophrenia. Similarly, many anti-depressants 'work' by elevating the level of serotonin in the brain, but we have little idea how serotonin is involved with depression, or even what depression really is. In the case of Lithium, we are not sure either how or why it works.

Everybody blithely ignores these problems because the real engine behind this development is economic. A 1991 study estimated that bipolar disorder—just one diagnosable condition—cost America 45 billion dollars in lost productivity and cost of care or incarceration.[45] That is the scale of the problem. But in seeking a solution, governments tend to focus on the lowest cost: pills are much cheaper than asylums or lengthy psychoanalysis or psychotherapy. The effective definition of a 'cure' has become that it makes a person less burdensome to the state and more able to provide for themselves economically, so the psychiatric profession and the state conspire to control the mad. These developments greatly extended the scope in psychiatry and therefore its power. Psychiatry can create a diagnosis wherever they can prescribe a pill, and diagnoses expanded to include all the marginal cases that previously were dismissed as mild eccentricities. In effect, what a diagnosis actually is has shifted: the doctor is merely identifying in the patient the symptom that a particular drug counteracts. That is a 'cure' of a pattern of behaviour that was never understood in the first place.

It was scepticism of these developments that led to the birth of the anti-psychiatry movement in the 1960s. Szasz was the major theoretician in this field. He earned himself notoriety and the total condemnation of his own profession with this opening of his most famous book:

Psychiatry is conventionally defined as a medical specialty concerned with the diagnosis and treatment of mental diseases. I submit that this definition, which is still widely accepted, places psychiatry in the company of alchemy and astrology and commits it to the category of pseudoscience.[46]

The Myth of Mental Illness by Szasz was published in 1961 in the same year as Foucault's *The History of Madness*. But the idea that madness is a social construct without any scientific justification had been around for a while before that. Psychiatry to date has been pre-scientific, and without an explanatory theory of causality, it has been difficult for its critics to attack it in a systematically scientific way. For example, much of Szasz's criticism of Freud as being unscientific resulted from him cherry-picking Freud's least scientific statements. Let me demonstrate that this approach is questionable, by doing the same to him:

> I submit that the concept of a distinctively human, normal or well-functioning personality is rooted in psychosocial and ethical criteria. It is not biologically given, nor are biological determinants especially significant for it. ... Hence I eschew biological considerations as explanations, and instead try to construct a consistently moral and psychosocial explanatory scheme.[47]

Szasz wrote that. But you could be forgiven for guessing that it was written by Freud, Charcot, Jung or pretty much any other theoretician from the last century or so. What is the science of morality? It is not very clever saying psychiatry is unscientific if you do not have a more scientific alternative of your own.

Szasz had his impact, and much of his criticism of psychiatry is still valid half a century after *The Myth of Mental Illness* first appeared. But the anti-psychiatry movement, like all other movements in the field, ultimately burnt out, because it too provided no alternative theory. It was a deconstruction without a reconstruction. Today we continue to flip between psychotherapy and psychopharmacology, neurological and psychological theories, chemical cures and talking cures.

Worst of all, we have a steady drift back towards incarceration as a means of managing the mad. The apparent untreatable nature of many personality disorders is leading to despair within the communities of practitioners who aim to help people with such conditions. One author concluded a 200-page book on psychopathy by joking that the shortest chapter was the one on treatment.[48] It is a reflection on how little psychiatry has achieved that we are returning to practices that we knew were hopeless in the nineteenth century. For instance, Rikers Island is a vast prison complex just off New York City. Almost 4,000 (40 per cent) of its prisoners have mental illnesses[49] and this, astonishingly, is as many as all the patients in all the mental hospitals in New York State.[50] These numbers are spiralling upward, as is the violence and repression used in controlling them—truly a return to discredited practices of two centuries ago. The transfer of responsibility for managing the mad from the medical profession to the prison service was completely unplanned. It was neither the policy of any political administration, nor was it based on scientific or medical advice, and the prison service certainly did not volunteer for the task. Organisations like the American Psychiatric Association (APA) spend their days pretending that consensus is emerging, where really opinions remain just as divided. We now have a world where it seems normal to suppose that everybody has something wrong with them.

Above all this, Big Pharma has the last laugh. In the 1960s, the tranquillizer Valium (diazepam) became the world's most widely prescribed drug. Antidepressants such as Prozac (fluoxetine) are among the most profitable drugs, and the marketing genius of these drugs is that people demand them from their doctors; sometimes even going as far as faking symptoms to achieve this. Doctor-prescribed narcotics does not get you a prison sentence like possession of cocaine, and some doctors in America will give you a prescription on demand for a fee. In some American states, this is not even illegal, which creates the situation of drug tourism, where people will cross a state border to obtain a prescription-high[51] that is unavailable in their home state. Today, three out of the ten most profitable drugs are for treating psychiatric conditions, and antidepressants are the most profitable drug sector after heart disease medication.[52] One in seven American children is diagnosed as having 'attention deficit hyperactivity disorder (ADHD)' and the doctor–patient role is reversed as parents beg doctors to diagnose ADHD in their naughty children so that they can medicate them with Ritalin (methylphenidate) for an easier life. This occurs despite the fact that there is absolutely no scientific evidence that ADHD is even a medical condition—it is merely a collection of all the things about children that adults do not like. The stigma of mental illness has been largely eradicated. Yet we still have no idea what it actually is.

THE START OF A NEW THEORY

A human is the only animal that can out-think its own biology. Emotions are biological action drivers and when humans try to out-think them, they no longer promote survival in the way that evolution by natural selection would dictate. This leads to self-destructive actions. Psychology only exists because a human can perform a self-destructive action. When a thirsty person drinks or a humiliated person lashes out at their persecutor, this is not explained by psychology; it is explained by evolutionary biology. If we can explain logically why a person might do something that cannot be explained by evolutionary biology, then we are tackling the questions of 'psychology' in a novel way. I am trying neither to refute psychology nor to rewrite it, since this would in any case be impossible to do without understanding it. But in trying to demonstrate that we can account for everything a human does using just evolutionary theory and logic, I am effectively questioning the very need for psychology. I can do this without even bothering to study it.

Foucault concludes *The History of Madness* with this passage:

> In our naivety, we perhaps imagined that we had described a psychological type, the madman, across 150 years of his history. But we are forced to admit that in writing this history of the mad, what we have done – not on the level of a chronology of discoveries, or

a history of ideas, but by following the links in the chain of the fundamental structures of experience – is to write the history of the things that made possible the very appearance of a psychology. And by that we understand a cultural fact peculiar to the Western world since the nineteenth century: this massive postulate defined by modern man, but which also defines him in return – *human beings are not characterised by a certain relationship to truth; but they contain, as rightly belonging to them, a truth that is simultaneously offered and hidden from view.*

. . . *Homo psychologicus* (psychological man) is descended from *homo mente captus* (insane man). As the only language that can speak is that of alienation, psychology is therefore only possible in the criticism of man or the criticism of itself.[53]

This argument agrees with my whole approach in this and my previous book. Foucault continues:

The world believes that madness can be measured, and justified by means of psychology, and yet it must justify itself when confronted by madness. . . And nothing within itself, and above all nothing that it can know of madness, serves to show that these oeuvres of madness prove it right.[54]

I neither agree with Szasz that 'mental illness' is a myth, nor with Foucault that it is a social construct, nor with the widely accepted psychiatric doctrine that it is a disease of either a physico-chemical or neurobiological nature. Proponents of psychiatry point out how stable psychiatric diagnoses have been over time—sometimes for centuries—and this is evidence of a real psychopathological structure; but I demonstrate that this is due to a finite number of *logical* mechanisms—each distinct—that give rise to separate conditions of madness.

Simple self-destruction, of which all of us are guilty in small part, is rationally derived from misunderstandings of emotions. This misunderstanding is derived from the fact that we pretend with our emotional behaviour. Madness is simply caused by compounded pretending with behaviour, resulting in misunderstandings of emotions of a more complex nature. I describe these compound misunderstandings and demonstrate that each mechanism causes different patterns of repetitive self-destructive action. Psychiatrists through the ages have been astute in spotting the differences between these mechanisms, even though they may not understand the structure of the mechanisms themselves.

A human is a robustly logical computational device that has the additional complexity of being able to self-reference: a human can impersonate its own behaviour. This leads to the possibility of circular causality and, as any computer scientist knows, this can have unusual and unintended consequences. If a self-destructive action is rational, then we can combine elements of self-destructiveness together to create self-destructive actions of a compound nature operating at a higher level of complexity.

In this way, we can construct models of human actions that are pure logical hypotheses, and once we have explored all the possibilities, we can start to ask ourselves whether these models appear to simulate the human conditions that psychiatrists call 'mental disorders'. At that point, we will have a scientific hypothesis that gives scientists studying in this field a new basis for interpreting their findings. I demonstrate that explanations all start dropping neatly into place like jigsaw pieces. If the scientific community largely agrees with me, then consensus will grow that this model really does describe how these conditions actually work. If that occurs, the very concept of 'madness' joins 'psychology' in the ether of forgotten notions.

It is the thesis of this book that madness, like everything else that a human does, is rational. A human tries to out-think its own emotions, which is a form of self-reference that leads to unusual consequences. Even human actions that are judged to be mad are logically derived from a particular combination of behavioural inputs.

A HUMAN AS A COMPUTATIONAL MACHINE

Philosophers have rather particular ideas about how science ought to be done, but scientists tend to ignore this and do just what they fancy. However, by a coincidental convergence of thinking, theoretical physicists do science almost exactly the way that philosophers think is proper. This is quite strange because physicists tend not to be particularly philosophically aware, mainly because the philosophical foundations of their science have not really shifted since the time of Isaac Newton and so they do not think about it that much. Their method is more or less as follows: generate a hypothetical mathematical model of how the universe works, and demonstrate that the model is self-consistent and reflects how the previously observed universe actually does work. The model is then extrapolated beyond what has been seen before to make wider predictions of how the universe ought to work—assuming that the model is actually correct. This extrapolation is the driver of experimentation. The experiments start with devising ways of observing phenomena that have not been seen before, and when the model correctly predicts the outcome of the experiment, theoretical physicists all dance a merry jig. If it does not, they scrap the model and start over again. For example, Albert Einstein correctly predicted the rate at which light ought to bend when passing through a gravitational field, although nobody had previously even considered this possibility. Another instance is the Higgs boson, a hypothetical particle that is purely the extrapolated prediction of a model of particle physics; so physicists dig tunnels under the Alps to demonstrate that it actually exists. The Large Hadron Collider is demonstrating that the mathematical model of particle physics that has dominated thinking in recent decades is most likely correct.

Psychologists think that they cannot work this way and, consequently, philosophers have a suspicion that they are not proper scientists. There were lots of philosophers around the middle of the twentieth century who made snotty remarks about the scientific credentials of psychologists. The major figures on this list would include Gilbert Ryle, a British philosopher who said, when inquiring into the nature of psychology, that 'the right answer to the question seems to be that the abandonment of the dream of psychology as a counterpart to Newtonian science';[55] Ludwig Wittgenstein, who said that he could not see how psychologists' experimental methodology could be really sound if they are unable to see a thought;[56] and Popper, who blasted Freud with both barrels.[57] These criticisms of psychology never went away. But philosophers went a bit quiet on the subject out of embarrassment: they got lost in their own ridiculous discussions about the 'mind' and 'free will', and ultimately it turned out that they had none of the answers either. Even if you think that psychology *is* a mature science, you would be hard pressed to describe their methodology as succinctly as I just described that of physics.

In *The Logic of Self-Destruction*, I attempted to tackle the problems of psychology the way that a theoretical physicist would, i.e. as a partisan philosopher, the right way. In *Part I: The Human Algorithm*, I demonstrated that we could generate a model of how a human worked that could account for all human actions (including the self-destructive ones). And in *Part II: Irrefutable Thoughts*, I built models of ideologies and religions (including Nazism and fictitious religions). I tried to demonstrate that all these oddities occurred because humans are self-referencing machines that impersonate their own behaviour.

Theoretical physicists achieve great things only because they have at their disposal a huge arsenal of powerful mathematics. Einstein, for example, would have been unable to produce his theories of relativity unless Muhammad Al-Khwarizmi had given us algebra in the eighth century, and Newton (or was it Gottfried Wilhelm Leibniz?) had given us calculus in the seventeenth century. Einstein used very old mathematics to solve problems that had only recently been realised.

To convert psychology into a robust science, we need to develop the necessary mathematics. An emotion is a biological thermostat. A thermostat triggers a sequence of events when a set of circumstances pertains: when it is sufficiently cold, it switches on your heating system. Hunger is a thermostat that switches on your searching-for-food routine when your stomach is sufficiently empty. When your stomach is full it switches it off again. Pity is a thermostat that switches on your helping-someone-in-difficulty routine and, when they are no longer in difficulty, it switches off again. Anger switches on when other people fail to fulfil their social obligations, and guilt switches on when other people point out that we have failed to fulfil our own social obligations. Guilt and anger both switch off when everybody is fulfilling their proper duty, so together guilt and anger acts as a mechanism to regulate our social interactions. Each emotion is a biological function that converts a set of circumstances into a particular action state.[58]

The extraordinary range of human actions, together with their apparent randomness, has caused many thinkers over the last three millennia to speculate about human action being caused by 'free will'. But nobody has ever set out how this would work in a form that a scientist would recognise as a hypothesis. After a couple of millennia of philosophical debate, we have reached this moment of epic stalemate: proponents of 'free will' cannot tell us what it *is*, and proponents of 'determinism' cannot tell us how it *works*.

There have been other supposed explanations of the apparent randomness and occasionally self-destructive nature of human action. For example, Freud essentially argued that if a human could perform a self-destructive action, then there must be something wrong with the brain's algorithm. He claimed that the unconscious mind causes us to perform irrational actions. I set out to demonstrate that a human action is not chosen; it is calculated. The brain algorithm that performs this calculation does not have a problem with it. It works just fine, and we could deduce a model for it that is self-consistent. The possibility of a self-destructive action is not due to a problem with the algorithm, but problems with the input to the algorithm—namely that humans perform tactical deception with their emotional behaviour.

To achieve this, I have had to show that there is 'mathematics' to how a human works. In an animal, an emotion drives an action, but a human (who can conceive of a future emotion) calculates an action to achieve an emotional goal. To do this optimally, they have to be able to correctly identify their own emotions and understand what causes them. A concept of an emotion is a derivative of behaviour. Darwin demonstrated in *The Expression of Emotions in Man and Animals*[59] that emotional behaviour was universal among humans, as was our ability to recognise and interpret it. In other words, an Aboriginal Australian and an Amazonian Indian would recognise and correctly identify each other's facial expressions upon first meeting.

Several philosophers, including Wittgenstein, deduced that our ability to have a word for an emotion is purely because the behaviour is on display. Without the behaviour, I cannot know that you experience the emotion and you cannot know that I experience it, so we could not have a word for it because we would have no common reference point. The word for an emotion therefore does not reference a feeling, as most people would consider. Strictly speaking, it references whatever is the cause of the behaviour, and the feeling is merely hypothesised. It is usual to presume that the feeling underlies the emotion itself, but when the behaviour has been modified by a tactical deception, this presumption is no longer correct. What causes the behaviour would be the cause of the tactical affectation. In the case of tactical suppression, the behaviour is absent, and with it, the means of identifying the emotion.

A human's understanding of his or her own emotions is therefore derived from behaviour, and tactical deception with that behaviour causes that understanding to be incorrect. Calculating an action to achieve an emotional goal, where the concept of the emotion is incorrect, results in a self-destructive action. There is nothing irrational about this, and the idea of 'irrationality' is scientifically incoherent and the product of some pretty sloppy thinking on the part of some of history's greatest thinkers.

Sadly, I was forced to stop short of explaining how we could use the model to drive an experimental programme, so the theory is just not as neat as theoretical physics. The fundamental difficulty, for a scientist, is figuring out whether biology causes a particular unit of observable emotional behaviour, or whether it is caused by a human out-thinking its biology. The model therefore remains within the realm of philosophy, and is merely a scientific hypothesis until a proper scientist (i.e. not me) figures out a way of demonstrating experimentally that the model is actually correct—or not, as the case might be.

In *The Logic of Self-Destruction*, I described in *Part I: The Human Algorithm* how a human logically derives a self-destructive action in the abstract. Then, I explained in *Part II: Irrefutable Thoughts* that all ideological and religious beliefs were actually logical tautologies that would ultimately become destructive to the people who believed them. In this book, I am going to extrapolate these ideas to higher levels of complexity to demonstrate that we can rationally derive self-destructive action states that are also of greater complexity. These are observable in humans, and we sometimes call it madness.

Doctors have persuaded us that they should handle these problems—not logicians—so they became known as 'mental illnesses', until it became apparent that maybe they were not illnesses at all, at which point they became known as 'mental disorders'. Despite this, we still think that physicians are best qualified to deal with these particular human problems. If belief systems are logical and so is madness, then it seems reasonable to consider that belief systems that have the characteristics of madness are also logical. In this way, I intend to demonstrate in a future book that madness can go viral throughout a society to produce what I call 'annihilationist' ideologies like the Islamic State in Iraq and Syria, Boko Haram, the Lord's Resistance Army and Nazism.

A logical human computes the path of least resistance through a maze of data about their environment that is replete with fallacies. Most of these fallacies become apparent when information contradicts them. But pretended behaviour is a falsehood that leads to a self-destructive action, the origin of which is rarely apparent. Beliefs have an impact on this in that a person's ideology or religion is central to everything that they think and do, and is on one level irrefutable to them and on another a contradiction, in that it defeats their own self-interest. These are some of the most difficult problems of humanity, but they arise because humans are individually self-referencing mechanisms, and humanity is collectively a self-referencing mechanism. They do this in a number of ways, but I have been focusing on one way, namely that they impersonate their own and each other's behaviour. A mechanism that self-references is likely to sprout circular causality. This is difficult to interpret scientifically, and we can only really understand it by thinking about it as a mathematical problem.

My work is to demonstrate that humans are robustly logical computational devices. Self-destructive actions are rational, so are beliefs; the psychiatric conditions that the common man calls madness are rational, and so are annihilationist ideologies. If I can demonstrate all that, I will have completed my mission. Nothing is irrational—not even madness or fundamentalism! Once we accept this, we can finally take the concept of irrationality and put it in the same trash can where we previously put the concepts of the soul, the unconscious mind and free will.

To claim that 'mental disorders' are logical is a radical new way of thinking about the problem. I am constructing these hypothetically by using combinations of emotional misconception, predicting what patterns of actions will be deduced from such a situation and then comparing that with how psychiatrists observe known mental disorders as they appear from the outside. Previously, there was almost no theory about how these worked as mechanisms. Since there is no theory of causality, that means there are no experts, so there is absolutely no reason why some random logician like myself cannot address the issue.

Scientists who study mental disorders have approached the problem from the perspective of psychology, sociology and neuroscience, but recent research has focused on finding ways that mental illnesses are correlated with brain abnormalities. This enables scientists to surmise that the disorder is caused by the abnormality, but it does not give many clues about how it actually functions. My approach is the opposite of this one. I start by making a sweeping simplifying assumption: I assume that everybody has a 'normal' brain (whatever *that* is). This means that I am constructing a model of how a human works that assumes that a human brain is a constant—in effect I am ignoring brain abnormalities. Before we can figure out what a human brain does, we have to establish what a human is *for*, in other words, what is its objective. This is a philosophical question, not a scientific one.

We could regard a really destructive ideology like Nazism to be a form of mass-psychopathic personality disorder; yet it is safe to assume that the entire German nation did not have a correlated brain abnormality. In *Part II: Irrefutable Thoughts* of *The Logic of Self-Destruction*, it was necessary for me to demonstrate how normal people could believe in Nazism en masse.[60] I explained the extremities of ideology, while making an assumption of believers with normal brains. And here I seek to do the same thing for a 'mental disorder' in an individual. In other words, my aim is to demonstrate that a person without a brain abnormality can have an apparent mental disorder that is entirely logical in its structure.

We can hypothesise a logical structure for a mental disorder without worrying ourselves about the complications of how that works at a neurological level. Noam Chomsky demonstrated that language was generated algorithmically, and he concluded that these algorithms must be encoded in the brain. However, worrying about how this all works at a neurological level was simply not a part of Chomsky's project, so he left that to other people to figure out. I am similarly concerned with the conceptual architecture of thought and not its bioelectronics. My work is to demonstrate that all human actions are the product of a brain algorithm, and I am now going to extrapolate that algorithm to cover actions that we have historically described as being mad.

I hope that neuroscientists will not think that I am criticising their work. But it is my contention that until we can form an understanding of how madness functions in a normal brain, we have no hope of understanding it with the added complication of a brain abnormality. The smart way to solve a problem is the simplest way. Figuring out the impact of brain abnormalities is not a scientific error, but a strategic one, since it involves trying to understand the really difficult cases before we have mastered the simple ones. This is like attempting to climb Mount Everest by the North Face without ropes or oxygen, when you have never gone up the 'easy' way with a string of Sherpas pulling you along.

THE THEORETICAL STARTING POINT

Let me summarise the theory of *Part I: The Human Algorithm* of *The Logic of Self-Destruction*, since this is the foundation from which I will be working.[61] A biological emotion is a product of evolution by natural selection. I define an emotion as a biological mechanism that converts a stimulus into a conscious urge to perform an action that enhances biological fitness. This urge is variable depending upon the severity of the circumstances; so the longer an animal waits since it last ate, the urge to seek food that we call 'hunger' becomes stronger. The circumstances that an animal faces will generally involve compound stimuli. For example, a dog might face both danger and an empty stomach. Fear and hunger will each have a value for the dog and depending upon these relative values, the dog might forgo the meal and run away, grab the food and then run away, or eat the food with a cautious eye on the proximate threat. This is clearly something that the dog probably does not have a choice about, since a dog just reacts and cannot second-guess that reaction.

In every circumstance, the animal has to compute the course of action that optimises biological fitness—the optimal strategy to ensure survival, reproduction and survival of offspring to maximise the propagation of its genes into the next generation. However, animals cannot do mathematics, so biology provides them with a computational substitute: each emotion returns a value based upon circumstances, and the animal acts according to the emotion with the highest value at that moment. That might seem like a base objective, but animals that do not operate that way do not propagate their genes, and so we do not have to trouble ourselves about wondering about what they are like, because they do not exist. This is how evolution by natural selection works: the animal with the instinctive strategies that maximise the transmission of its genes has the most offspring.

I divide emotions into four main groups: (1) basic survival: fear, hunger, thirst, etc.; (2) reproductive: lust, jealousy, humiliation and love of offspring; (3) social: guilt, pity, anger and gratitude; and (4) strategic: anxiety, regret and sadness. I intentionally left out happiness. Readers of *Part I: The Human Algorithm* of *The Logic of Self-Destruction* will recall that I speculate that happiness is a form of invented emotion, so does not have an evolutionary origin at all.[62] Life that is a product of evolution by natural selection does not have a purpose beyond survival and reproduction. Social interactions, such as playfulness, only exist because social mechanisms themselves have origins in the evolution of survival mechanisms. Only humans realise this, and the urge to invent a purpose is the origin of beliefs and religions. Along those lines, I have also intentionally left out romantic love. Emotions are transient and love endures, so love is a belief rather than an emotion. Part of the reason for this confusion, is that it is a belief about an emotion.

Of the above list, all of these emotions are present in chimpanzees, with the probable exception of what I call the strategic emotions. Chimpanzees almost certainly have limited concepts of abstract space and time and therefore, cannot spend hours thinking about hypothetical or future threats. Philosophers at least as far back as Jean-Jacques Rousseau have doubted that animals experience anxiety, and Søren Kierkegaard said: 'Time does not really exist without unrest; it does not exist for dumb animals who are entirely without anxiety.'[63] When we go a little further back down the evolutionary path, we find that fewer of these emotions are present. For example, I think it is demonstrable that chimpanzees have guilt, but doubtful that dogs do. What dog owners think is guilty behaviour when they scold their pet, is almost certainly behaviour associated with subservience. Probably the oldest emotions are lust and the basic survival emotions, and we can see the evolutionary origins of these in the simplest of non-vertebrate animals. Solitary reptiles and amphibians probably have no other emotions.

It makes most sense to consider an emotion in a social mammal to be a function that has two separate outputs: on the one hand, we have the urge to adopt an action state; on the other we have an expression of that urge that is a means of communication between animals of the same social group. This is essential to the functioning of the social group, since they not only know what each is doing, but why they are doing it. We could explain it diagrammatically in Figure 1 as follows:

FIGURE 1: DIAGRAM OF A GENERIC BIOLOGICAL EMOTION

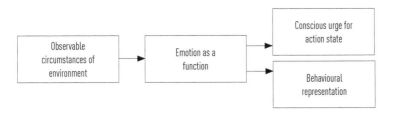

Darwin understood the evolutionary origins of the basic survival and reproductive emotions and he explained the evolutionary mechanisms well in *On the Origin of the Species*[64] and *The Descent of Man.*[65] He then went on to study emotional expression in some detail in his final major book, *The Expression of Emotions in Man and Animals.*[66] But he did not know what a gene was and, although he recognised that emotional expression was universal and therefore social emotions probably had an evolutionary origin, he was unable to describe the evolutionary mechanism. We had to wait until 1964, when W. D. Hamilton published *The Genetical Evolution of Social Behaviour,*[67] before we began to understand the mechanism for the evolution of social emotions.

Let me explain briefly their evolutionary origin. Hunger drives the action of seeking food and this is essential to survival in an individual animal. Pity drives the action of assisting another animal that is in difficulty. Each of these enhances the biological fitness of the individual that acts on that emotional driver. In other words, it increases the chances that the actor's genes will be carried forward to the next generation. In comparison, the evolutionary origin of pity is a little more complicated than hunger because it operates along two separate pathways. Firstly, we have to look at how pity works in family groups—so-called 'nepotistic altruism'. Acting on pity towards your sibling enhances your biological fitness because your sibling carries many of the same genes as yourself and evolution selects at the gene level. The probability that your sibling obtained a particular gene from the same ancestor is 100 per cent for your identical twin, 50 per cent for your full sibling and 25 per cent for your half sibling. Evolutionary theorists call these percentages, the degree of 'relatedness'. Pity, when applied to your sibling, increases the chance that your genes survive and will be passed to the next generation through your sibling's progeny. A demonstration of how nepotistic altruism works can be seen in monkey troupes, where a monkey will groom another troupe member with a frequency that is roughly proportional to that monkey's degree of relatedness.

Secondly, we need to consider non-nepotistic pity. This benefits the actor if the beneficiary has genes for reciprocity, and this is almost certainly the case in most social vertebrates. We might say that nepotistic pity and non-nepotistic pity are separate emotions, and they probably have separate evolutionary origins. But they have become almost impossible to separate, so we tend to consider them to be the same thing. Pity, sympathy and gratitude all drive altruistic actions, and shame inhibits antisocial actions. Together, these form a mechanism that regulates the actions of animals that function in advanced social groups in such a way as to enhance biological fitness.

It is important to remember that this works at the level of the gene. It might appear to operate at the level of the social group, but this only appears to be the case because a successful gene replicates from one generation to another and eventually finds its way into all individuals in the social group. What looks like a group phenomenon, is actually individual phenomena that all individuals share because they all share certain common genes.

To understand how deep these evolutionary origins are, we need to study chimpanzees. It is astonishing how similar to us they are. These are the observations of the primatologist Frans de Waal:

> The playface, the grin, and the begging gesture are not imitations of human behaviour, but natural forms of nonverbal communication that humans and chimpanzees have in common. Some unusual signals, such as the way Mama shakes her head to say no, may very well be the result of human influence. But even this very special signal was observed by Adriaan Kortlandt among wild chimpanzees.[68]

Almost all human emotions can be observed in chimpanzees, which should not be shocking since we have common ancestors. Once again, this is the observation of de Waal:

> Humans are talking primates, but in fact their behaviour is not very different from that of chimpanzees. People engage in verbal fights, provocative or impressive word displays, protesting interruptions, conciliatory remarks, and many other patterns of verbal activity that chimpanzees perform without an accompanying text. When humans resort to actions instead of words the resemblance is even greater. Chimpanzees scream and shout, bang doors, throw objects, call for help, and afterward they may make up by a friendly touch or embrace. We humans also display all these patterns, usually without taking a conscious decision to do so, and maybe our motives are not so very different from those of chimpanzees.[69]

In humans, the simple mechanism of emotions driving actions undergoes a fatal twist. Humans have language, and this enables them to form concepts of future emotion. Only in a few other smart animals is there any evidence that they have a concept of their own behaviour, and there is little evidence that other animals can plan or have a concept of a future. Chimpanzees provide important evidence here because it appears that they *do* understand the future and *can* plan, but only over short-term horizons—perhaps up to an hour or so. Some biologists are sceptical that animals can foresee the future at all, but chimpanzees have a farewell routine when they are about to part company, and this can only take place with a mutual awareness of a future event—albeit one that will occur within a few minutes. However, chimpanzees are clearly highly intelligent animals and the difficulty that they have stretching their concept of future beyond this makes it clear just how remarkable a human's conception of the future really is. A 25-year-old human can open a retirement plan or take out a mortgage, and by doing so they are planning further into the future than the entire span of their life to date. A human who arranges his finances to avoid inheritance tax is planning for a future beyond their grave. If concepts of future and concepts of behaviour are both difficult for animals to grasp, then we can be confident that planning future emotional states is unique to humans.

In humans, the emotion does not drive the action. Instead, we calculate the action to strategise a future emotion. For example, an animal only seeks food when it is hungry, but humans seek food in advance to avoid hunger—without this capability, we would not yet have invented agriculture. Thus, we reverse the causality of an action: in an animal the emotion pushes the action, but in a human the action is calculated to pull the emotion. The emotion in a human is still a product of evolution by natural selection, and so strategising the future emotion will still drive a survival-enhancing action if we do the calculation correctly. However, this will not be the case if we have a misconception about the identity of the emotion or what causes it. This would be unusual in the case of hunger (the exception being people with eating disorders—more on that later!), so we correctly deduce the action to strategise its avoidance. This can no longer be presumed to be the case when we are considering emotions where we perform tactical deception with the behaviour.

Once again, studying chimpanzees is key in reaching this conclusion. A chimpanzee can only perform tactical manipulation of emotional behaviour at the margin: they can suppress emotional behaviour by manipulating their face with their fingers. In contrast, humans can do this fluidly and effortlessly. There is documented evidence of apparent tactical deception in intelligent animals such as primates, squirrels and crows, but little of this has been peer-reviewed by philosophers. As an example, nobody has a problem with the idea that a squirrel burying nuts has the effect of knowing that winter is coming without the squirrel actually knowing that winter is coming. It should therefore be easy for us to consider that a squirrel's action that has the effect of tactical deception might involve no understanding of that deception. Most of the apparent cases of tactical deception in animals could be interpreted as being behaviour that has the *effect* of tactical deception without the animal having the *intent*. This is a philosophical question for which the answer is not clear. In any case, I can find no evidence in the scientific literature of animals seeming to tactically affect emotional behaviour. Tactical deception can be divided into four quadrants (2x2 matrix): action, non-action, affect and suppress, as seen in Table 1:

TABLE 1: INTENTION OF TACTICAL DECEPTION WITH EMOTIONAL BEHAVIOUR

Deception → Intended Response ↓	Affect	Suppress
Action: Make you do something	A car salesman pretends the customer is his friend to make them buy the car. Not buying the car feels like an act of betrayal.	When a man and woman have just met and each knows the other is attracted to them, the woman pretends to ignore the man to make him approach her.
Non-action: Stop you doing something	A parent pretends to be angry to stop a child stealing from the cookie jar.	Suppress excitement at having found something to prevent others rushing to claim it.

I believe that most tactical deception in the animal kingdom belongs in the bottom-right quadrant. Affectation of emotional behaviour is a more complex cognitive capability than suppression, because it requires a memory of both the behaviour and the response. There should, however, remain some philosophical doubt that some animals might do this with such conviction that they even fool animal behaviour researchers, but this is a stretch of the scientific imagination. It is also quite a complicated deception to make another do something advantageous to you by manipulating your behaviour, since this requires a very good understanding of proactive responses.

Humans perform tactical deception with emotional behaviour almost constantly. You might affect happiness and suppress anxiety because you think this makes you admired by your peers. The suppression of emotional behaviour disrupts our ability to correctly identify our emotions, and the affectation of emotions gives rise to a false understanding of what causes them. Thus, the prerequisites of our mechanism for deriving a survival-enhancing action are corrupted and the action is suboptimal. In this way, self-destructive actions are logically derived from misconstrued concepts of emotion, and these in turn are derived from emotional behaviour that is subject to tactical deception.

Most people would not consider hunger to be an emotion. However, hunger and pity are both what we would usually call feelings. Each feeling drives an action that is appropriate to it. That is the point—what it is *for*; so from my perspective there really is no difference. Hunger or needing to urinate have an apparent distinction from pity in that they seem less complicated, but I surmise that this has got more to do with the fact that we rarely have a reason to perform any tactical deception with the feelings of hunger or needing to urinate. An emotion is therefore only distinct from other feelings that drive action in that we get confused about it as a result of the tactical deception. I cannot see any other reason to regard them as fundamentally distinct.

When we compare emotions in humans and chimpanzees, the

comparison is difficult because tactical deception makes emotions hard to understand in humans. We need to look at chimpanzees to understand how they are supposed to work. For example, the emotion of anger evolved as a means of punishing cheaters, but this is difficult to see in humans because we commonly suppress it. But it can be observed in chimpanzees, as this passage from de Waal describes:

> This happened once after Puist had supported Luit in chasing Nikkie. When Nikkie later displayed at Puist she turned to Luit and held out her hand to him in search of support. Luit, however, did nothing to protect her against Nikkie's attack. Immediately Puist turned on Luit, barking furiously, chased him across the enclosure, and even hit him. If her fury was in fact the result of Luit's failure to help her after she had helped him, this would suggest that reciprocity among chimpanzees is governed by the same sense of moral rightness and justice as it is among humans.[70]

I am seeking to demonstrate that everything that is weird about humans stems from their ability to out-think their own biology. I am not totally inventing this idea, but the history of writing about emotion reveals a strange bifurcation of thinking between science and philosophy. Scientists since before Darwin have recognised that humans suppress emotion, and philosophers from Confucius to Rousseau have recognised that humans affect emotional behaviour. Confucius said: '... the forms of mourning observed without grief—these are things I cannot bear to see!'[71] The importance of this statement is that it makes it clear that humans have not only affected emotional behaviour since at least the fifth century BC, but they recognised that they were doing it—hence it was truly tactical. Before I wrote *The Logic of Self-Destruction*, I could not find anybody else who simultaneously examined both affectation and suppression, or anybody who considered that these deceptions have *logical* consequences.

Evolutionary theorists sometimes use a shorthand description of an animal as a 'survival machine', but the ability of a human to wilfully self-destruct makes this inappropriate. I capture this by changing the shorthand to reflect the inversion of the causality of an action in a human. We are 'machines that goal-seek emotional outcomes'. We calculate an action to achieve an emotional outcome, and the inputs to this algorithm are concepts of emotion derived from behaviour that may or may not be the subject of a behavioural manipulation.

Let us tabulate the ways that we can form a distorted concept of an emotion. There are two ways that we can perform a tactical deception with emotional behaviour: we can suppress it or we can affect it. And then we have to look at this from two perspectives: the first person and the second/third person, since it has a differing effect when the tactical deception is being performed by ourselves or by somebody else; so we can look at this as a simple binary model divided into four quadrants (2x2 matrix). Table 2 is a breakdown of the possible misconceptions of emotions where the tactical deception has become habitual:

TABLE 2: MISCONCEPTIONS OF EMOTIONS DUE TO HABITUAL TACTICAL DECEPTION

Effect on concept of the emotion	Affect	Suppress	
First person	You think you experience an emotion whether you do or not. However, the trigger for your affectation is understood by you to be a cause of the emotion. (For example, a salesman pretends to be excited about his product.)	You can identify the emotion in other people via the behaviour, but do not acknowledge that you experience it because your own behaviour is absent. (For example, a woman in an abusive relationship suppresses her fear of her partner.)	You have a correct concept of the emotion in other people, but an impaired ability to attribute the emotion to yourself.

Effect on concept of the emotion	Affect	Suppress	
Second/third person	You derive a false cause of the emotion. (For example, in America everybody pretends to be happy.)	The behavioural identifier is absent in other people; so when you encounter the emotion in yourself, if you guess its identity, you have no means of refuting the guess, so the guess sticks. (For example, in many Asian countries, everybody suppresses anger.)	You have an incorrect or absent concept of the emotion in others, and therefore cannot correctly identify it or its cause in yourself.
	False ideas of the cause of the emotion	Disruption of the ability to identify the emotion	

If a human is a machine that goal-seeks emotional outcomes, and they have a distorted idea of an emotion, we can deduce what the distorting effect will be on the action that such a person derives. Again, this forms a simple binary model divided into four quadrants (2x2 matrix) (Table 3):

TABLE 3: THE EFFECT ON HUMAN ACTION OF MISUNDERSTOOD EMOTIONS

Effect on the action	Affect	Suppress	
First person	You keep repeating an action you believe achieves an emotional outcome without being able to determine whether you were successful or not.	You cannot determine the action to achieve the emotional goal because you cannot identify the emotion in yourself.	You understand the emotional goal but cannot achieve it.
Second/third person	You perform an action that you think will achieve an emotional outcome, despite the fact that the emotional outcome is imagined.	You conclude that you have achieved an emotion; however, you may have misidentified it. This will lead to compulsion in the case of positive emotions and revulsion in the case of negative ones.	You cannot achieve the emotional goal, because you have false ideas of its cause or its identity.
	You think you know the action that achieves an emotional goal, but are mistaken.	You think you know the emotion that results from your action, but are mistaken.	

The matrices in Tables 2 and 3 are effectively elemental models of how a human calculates an action. They assume (unrealistically) that a human only has one emotion at a time; that the behavioural tactical deception is consistent and habitual, and that emotional objectives are based upon just one distinct emotion. That said, this is the way that all mathematical analysis is performed: start with atomic-level concepts and analyse the binary relations between such concepts. Once this is mastered, we can move on to molecular concepts and probabilistic relations.

Moving to a higher level of complexity does not stop it being a mathematical problem. Clearly, a human is multidimensional: his or her emotions cannot be easily distinguished and should be regarded as a sort of array; his or her emotional objectives are hybrid; and he or she lives in a world where tactical deception with emotional behaviour is varied but has notable correlations within family or cultural groups. For example, many Americans habitually pretend to be happy, but Eastern Europeans think that smiling too much means that you are stupid, so they have a correlated tendency to adopt the opposite behavioural tactical deception. Both of these deceptions have become so culturally embedded and so habitual that nobody thinks of them as deceptions anymore.

In *Part II: Irrefutable Thoughts* of *The Logic of Self-Destruction*, I looked at combining the first person and second/third person modules in the above matrices (Tables 2 and 3) in differing ways. I used this to build models of how ideologies and religions functioned. I demonstrated that they were logical in character and had the form of being logical tautologies in which a group of humans become ensnared. For example, I demonstrated that it could be logical to believe in a fictitious religion. Humans cannot find their way out of the tautology until a serendipitous event occurs to jolt them into a different perspective.

SELF-DESTRUCTION AND MADNESS – A CLEAR DISTINCTION

> A man who prefers to be dead rather than
> Red is normal. A man who says he has lost
> his soul is mad. A man who says that men are
> machines may be a great scientist. A man
> who says he is a machine is 'depersonalized'
> in psychiatric jargon. A man who says that
> Negroes are an inferior race may be widely
> respected. A man who says his whiteness is a
> form of cancer is certifiable.
> — R. D. Laing, The Divided Self[72]

Everybody performs self-destructive actions. You might smoke, procrastinate, or stay in a relationship or job that makes you miserable. All of these are self-destructive action states that are not considered mad. The approach in each edition of the DSM is often to state that a patient has such-and-such a disorder if they have four or more of the pertinent symptoms. This can lead to the easy misconception that one can be 35 per cent mad or 63 per cent mad. What I want to demonstrate is that madness is a clear discrete step from normal self-destruction. In a sense, this means that psychiatry is right in identifying a clear boundary. We could say that madness is self-destruction that is compulsive, repetitive or which continues long after it is abundantly clear that it is self-destructive. In Section B: Compulsions and Section C: Impulsions, I will demonstrate why compulsiveness or repetitiveness actually has a logical structure.

A self-destructive action is rationally derived when a human calculates an action to achieve an emotional outcome from a faulty understanding of that emotion. Misunderstandings of emotions are rationally derived from falsified behaviour that results from a tactical deception with such behaviour. That tactical deception arises because each individual is trying to get ahead of his or her peers, or at least be accepted by them. Pretending with your behaviour is simply a means for achieving this end. The swirling eddy that is humanity consists of everybody trying to get ahead, but collectively becoming the origin of everybody's self-destruction (including their own).

When we suppress behaviour, we disrupt the correct identification of emotions. When we affect it, we derive false understandings of what causes emotions. Madness, I hope to demonstrate, is what occurs when we combine these problems in complex patterns or when we make complex errors in the understanding of our emotions. This gives rise to concepts of emotion that are in compound error, leading to self-destruction of a higher order of complexity. This is not a continuum; it is a step-change in self-destructiveness.

Consider the following witness statement at a hypothetical murder trial: 'I saw the accused arriving at the victim's house at 10 p.m. on Tuesday.' This is a statement of fact, and like any other it can be in error (intentionally or otherwise). This statement has three elements: a person, a place and a time. But the statement could be in error about all three elements simultaneously: the witness saw somebody else who looked similar to the accused, arriving at the house next door to the victim's, at a time ten minutes after the murder took place, not before. In this case, the witness statement is in compound error.

To have an understanding of an emotion that is in compound error—namely, we are mistaken both about its identity and causality simultaneously—would require both suppression and affectation of emotional behaviour. This would appear to be contradictory if it occurred to one emotion according to one stimulus, since you cannot both pretend to be angry (for example) and suppress anger at the same time. However, we can achieve this situation if we approach it on the diagonal.

Consider a biological emotion 'E1' that is a biological function that turns the stimulus of circumstance 'C1' into the action state 'A1' and the behaviour state 'B1'. We could call C1 the 'Biological Stimulus' for the emotion E1 and represent it diagrammatically (Figure 2) like this:

FIGURE 2: DIAGRAM OF A GENERIC EMOTION

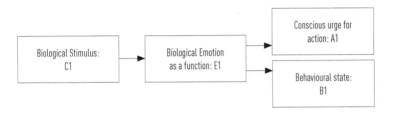

Now let us assume that when circumstance C1 arises, we suppress the behaviour B1 and simultaneously affect the behaviour associated with another emotion Ex—namely, we affect the behaviour Bx. C1, the Biological Stimulus for emotion E1, has therefore become the 'Affectation Stimulus' for the emotion Ex. Then we have created a situation of simultaneous suppression and affectation, but of two different emotional behaviours. We suppress the behaviour associated with E1 and affect that associated with Ex—both on the occurrence of a single stimulus C1. As an example, suppose that when someone experiences the Biological Stimulus that we associate with hunger, they suppress the hunger and affect shame, then they are simultaneously suppressing one emotion (hunger) and affecting another (shame)—both upon the occurrence of a single stimulus. I will explore this situation further in Section B: Compulsions. It is my contention that there are a finite number of ways that this situation can be established, and the rational consequences of this create a map of the spectrum of psychiatric disorders involving compulsive action states. Most of these fit the spectrum that psychiatrists used to call 'neurosis'.

In Section C: Impulsions, I will explore an alternative way that a human can form ideas of emotion that are in complex error. In particular, I want to examine what happens if a person is unable to identify two separate emotions in themselves because they grew up in an environment where the behaviour for both was suppressed. This gives rise to the possibility that they can identify these emotions the wrong way round. This has complex consequences in that a rational person in this situation will compute actions that other people consider inappropriate to their circumstances. I hope to demonstrate that this situation gives rise to the spectrum of psychiatric disorders that psychiatrists call 'acute personality disorder'. Readers of *Part II: Irrefutable Thoughts* of *The Logic of Self-Destruction*, will recall that I explained the Holocaust as a mechanism where humiliation was suppressed for a Biological Stimulus (namely, that hundreds of thousands of Germans, particularly children, died as a result of the blockade following World War I) and was replaced by a mythologised humiliation created by Hitler.[73] This resulted in a compulsive revenge response that did not have an identifiable target, so it went viral. Here, I will explore how a similar situation could occur in an individual human. I hope to demonstrate that the consequences of this can be explained, modelled and used as a map of acute personality disorders.

Finally, in Section D: Delusions, I will then consider whether it can also be rational to be psychotic. However, here I employ an argument that follows a completely separate line of reasoning from anything that I have considered elsewhere. This argument is centred around a different way in which a human can self-reference, and I use this idea to develop a hypothesis for a theory of psychosis as a mechanism.

This entire book assumes that a human is a robustly logical computational device. This does not of course *prove* that madness is rational, but it makes a compelling hypothesis from which scientists can contrive an experimental programme. Using pure theory, I can create a map of the range of mental disorders that we should expect to observe in humanity. And if my theoretical approach is considered reasonable by many researchers, then hopefully they would all start to interpret their results in this light. If I am correct, then hopefully their results will all lead to systematic and self-consistent explanations. And ultimately, this theoretical analysis will come to be *accepted* as science.

Only once we have mastered this does it make sense to return to looking at brain abnormalities to try to understand their impacts. In the psychiatry of the future, madness caused by brain abnormalities will surely be treated differently from madness that is rational. But by understanding why a particular rational structure might be emphasised by particular emotional qualities, we might then be able to understand why a particular individual is susceptible to a particular type of mental disorder, or why a particular form of madness runs in a family.

B:

COMPULSIONS

Aristotle is of the opinion all shame is for
some offence. But we find otherwise; it may
as well proceed from fear, from force and
inexperience, as vice; a hot liver; from a
hot brain, from wind, the lungs heated, or
after drinking of wine, strong drink,
perturbations, etc.
— Robert Burton, The Anatomy
of Melancholy[74]

A COMPULSION TO PERFORM AN ACTION

W.D. Hamilton, in my opinion, is the second most important evolutionary theorist after Darwin. However, he was not really a scientist at all, but a mathematician. My interest in him is that his methods were similar to my own—looking at scientific problems with a mathematician's hat on, and throwing in some thought experiments to make it all seem like certainty. But though he was a mathematician, today we think of him as a scientist, and this reveals something interesting about the distinction between mathematics and science: the boundary is fuzzy and it shifts. His mathematics morphed into science through no effort on his part.

Almost everything that Hamilton contributed to our understanding of evolution came about through mathematical and hypothetical reasoning. Hamilton demonstrated the importance of the concept of relatedness by explaining that evolution selects at the gene level, and 50 per cent of your genes were inherited by your full sibling from the same parent. Therefore, you should apply half as much effort into ensuring that your full sibling survives as for yourself. Hamilton's rule is that evolution selects for actions such that $C < r \times B$, where C is the cost of an action in terms of biological fitness, r is the degree of relatedness and B is the benefit in terms of biological fitness. Relatedness is a purely mathematical concept derived from probability theory. The concept of the evolutionarily stable strategy[75] is also a purely mathematical concept but derived instead from game theory. Hamilton used such concepts to engage in hypothetical reasoning that enabled him to create models for the evolution of altruism, spitefulness and other behavioural characteristics observed in the animal world.

W. D. Hamilton worked like a mathematician, but his theoretical output influenced the way that real scientists (that is field researchers) went about their work. Most of the scientific side of the evolutionary story came about when field researchers stumbled upon animals that had a particular characteristic that was determined by a single or very small number of individual genes. This makes them ideal for genetic experimentation. Gradually, they interpreted their experimental results in the light of Hamilton's hypothetical theories, and over time it became increasingly clear that everything that Hamilton had reasoned by thought experiment and mathematical modelling was absolutely right. At this point, Hamilton's work was no longer mathematics; it was science.

One of my favourite pieces of evolutionary research is the story of the 'hygienic bee'.[76] This is a species that throws diseased larvae out of the nest and thereby keeps the nest hygienic. But this behaviour is not found in all bee nests of the species. A researcher named W. C. Rothenbuhler found that when he crossed queens and drones of the hygienic and non-hygienic strain, he created a bee's nest that did not display the hygienic behaviour. Initially, he presumed that this was because the gene for the hygienic behaviour was recessive. But when he backcrossed the hybrid bees with the pure hygienic strain, he was very surprised by the result. He found that in the second generation hybrids, each bee nest was one of three distinct varieties: firstly, there were normal hygienic bees that expelled diseased larvae; secondly, there was a strain that was non-hygienic; and thirdly, there were half-and-half bees that opened up the cells of diseased larvae, but did not throw the larvae out. Rothenbuhler then opened the cells of the diseased larvae of the non-hygienic second strain and was amazed to find that the bees then threw out the larvae in the same way as the hygienic bees. Clearly, the only explanation for this is that there are just two genes that control this behaviour: one causes the bee to open up a cell in which a diseased larva lived, and the second causes the throwing out. The second strain only had the throwing-out gene, and the third only the opening-up gene.

This type of research is important because it makes it clear that it is perfectly fine to talk about genes *for* behaviour. These experiments also have a philosophical implication because they make it pretty clear that the bee does not know *what* it is doing and it does not know *why* it is doing it, which would seem to imply that a bee is just a biological robot. Since most of us assume that a bee does not have conscious experience, this is not really so odd. But these ideas eventually need to be extrapolated to more advanced animals— like humans.

Talking about genes *for* behaviour is a necessary step for my argument. When I say that most human emotions arose through evolution by natural selection, I am following a fairly orthodox evolutionary theorists' way of talking by speaking of a gene *for* sympathy or a gene *for* anger, even though the molecular reality at the level of DNA is almost certainly considerably more complex than that. Richard Dawkins explained in *The Extended Phenotype*[77] that it is fine to talk this way provided we understand that we should look at the genotype of an organism (such as a human) in a holistic way, and should stop thinking that DNA is like a string of beads where each bead is one gene that controls one characteristic. Mutation and crossing over can occur at any point, including in the middle of a hypothetical bead, and the characteristic might be determined by bits of DNA that might not all sit together on a chromosome.

Although neither Dawkins nor Hamilton talk much about human emotions, I do not think I would trouble either of them unduly if I was to speak about the gene *for* anger actually consisting of various bits of DNA scattered throughout a human (or chimpanzee) genome. Certain of these bits of DNA, in combination with others, would simultaneously be the gene *for* sympathy. I say this by way of preamble because I want to indulge in some hypothetical reasoning that involves playing fast and loose with all of these concepts at the same time.

I started with W. D. Hamilton because I wanted to compare what he did with what I am doing. I create logical models of how humans act, and this is pure hypothesis. I am not pretending that this is psychology; I am not even pretending that this is science. It would be wonderful if one day my hypothesis morphed into science and researchers all agreed that my way of looking at human nature was absolutely right. Alas, my hypothetical reasoning is more difficult than Hamilton's to convert into science. I am arguing that humans take the emotions that result from evolution by natural selection, and then employ tactical deception in the form of manipulating the behavioural characteristics that these genes should drive. For this theory to be turned into science in the same way as Hamilton's, we would need to find a human emotion that was driven by a single or very small number of genes, and then conduct experiments on people who did and did not have the gene. This seems an improbable situation; but even if we found such a thing, it would not be the end of our problems. We would then need to find an experimental method to determine whether a human's observable behaviour is driven by its biology or by a tactical affectation that results from it trying to out-think its biology. This, I suspect, is impossible.

In fact, the possibility of tactical deceptive portrayal of a form of emotional behaviour by people who do not have the gene for that behaviour is one reason why discovering the single gene for emotion is unlikely in the first place. Chairman Mao Zedong appeared to completely lack the moral emotions, but he was a consummate actor who could portray these emotions whenever the situation demanded.[78] To discover a biological emotion in a human that was controlled by a single gene, we would need to find one that bred pure in a Mendelian fashion,[79] and we can only spot this if the data is uncorrupted, i.e. not hiding behind a veil of behavioural manipulation.

Each of the four quadrants of Tables 2 and 3 (mentioned previously in Section A: Foundations – The Theoretical Starting Point), described a simple binary model of how a human can derive a self-destructive action. By combining these in different ways, we can hypothetically derive self-destructive actions of a more complex nature. I hope to demonstrate that some of these complex patterns of destructive actions bear similarities to 'mental disorders' and we can therefore construct a hypothesis, not only of what a 'mental disorder' is, but of how it actually works.

Let us imagine that there is a gene *for* each biological human emotion. This requires a conceptual leap because we are trapped by language into putting human emotions into buckets. We have separate words for pity and guilt, so we tend to think of those as two distinct emotions. This is clearly an unrealistic but necessary consequence of the way language works, so we need to amend this way of thinking. We should think of human emotions as forming a continuous multidimensional space, but none of us are much good at thinking multidimensionally. Let us therefore imagine that the genes *for* human emotions occur on a single continuous strip of DNA, and that human emotions form a continuum that parallels this strip. Each piece of the continuous DNA strip corresponds to a single piece on an emotional continuum. In following this line of thought, I do not think I am straying far from the methods of hypothetical reasoning that Dawkins and Hamilton employ. We could display this diagrammatically (Figure 3) as follows:

FIGURE 3: BIOLOGICAL EMOTIONS CODED IN HUMAN DNA

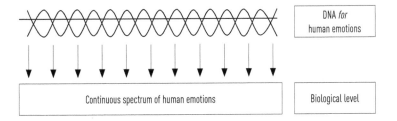

I use the 'Biological level' box to make the distinction between a biological emotion (that is found in your genes) and a concept of emotion (that exists in your brain because you understand the point of an emotion and can out-think your own biology). I use the term 'instinct' in a particularly technical way: I am using it to refer to actions that are driven by emotions without the intervention of tactical deception. There is nothing unusual about altering the meaning of a term to suit a technical need. Critics of evolutionary theory point out that Hamilton's brilliant description of the evolution of altruism uses the word 'altruism' in a confusing, non-standard way suited solely to supporting his theories: Hamilton is concerned with behaviour that has the *effect* of benefiting another, whereas humans tend to think that altruism's true sense is all about the *purpose*.[80] This criticism of Hamilton is irrelevant because the effect of altruism evolved before humans—who can out-think their own biology—understood why they were acting that way. Altruism started as an instinctive response, and ended intentional. My critics will no doubt say that I am using the term 'instinct' in a non-standard way suited solely to support my theory; and they would be right, but there is no problem with this if it is clear how I am using the word. I have previously argued that humans form concepts of their instinctive actions and then second-guess these actions.

This, of course, means that we can no longer call the resulting action instinctive—the action is driven by an idea of an emotion, not by a biological emotion itself. The idea of the emotion is a derivative of behaviour, and this might have been subjected to a tactical deception, so concept and biology part company. It is therefore probably meaningless to say that any human action (beyond infancy) is purely instinctive in the sense I use it here. Tactical deception of human emotional behaviour can become learned, and then habitual, and then the fact that the deception existed in the first place is forgotten. When this happens, a human's behaviour becomes cast in concrete, and that behaviour is *not* driven by a biological, instinctive emotion (and therefore that human's genes) but by a belief. The action is not driven genetically, but by a human out-thinking its biology.

So now we have to add an extra layer to our diagram (Figure 4). What happens when we add the layer that is a product of a well-seasoned tactical manipulation that now seems to be normal to the person portraying it?

FIGURE 4: GENERIC DRIVING EMOTIONS WITH SWITCHED BEHAVIOUR

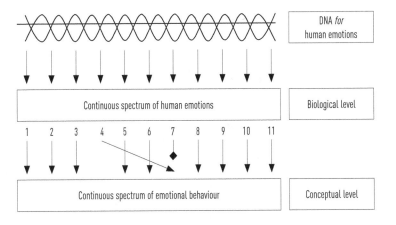

The diagram in Figure 4 is a model of a hypothetical individual who combines two forms of habitual behaviour manipulation: when they encounter the Biological Stimulus for emotion 4, they suppress the behaviour associated with that emotion and instead affect the behaviour of emotion 7. In other words, the Biological Stimulus for emotion 4 becomes the Affectation Stimulus for emotion 7. In this simple way, we have created a situation of simultaneous suppression and affectation of behaviour. However, it is displayed as a single behaviour associated with emotion 7 that occurs in circumstances different to the Biological Stimulus for emotion 7. They will have a concept of emotion 7 in themselves—because that is the behaviour they display—but no concept of emotion 4 ever occurring in themselves, because the behaviour is absent. This particular combination of emotional manipulation could be described thus: they are misidentifying emotion 4 in that they think it is emotion 7, and they are reinforcing this by affecting the behaviour associated with emotion 7.

Before we can analyse how such a person would act, we need to explore one essential point about how biological emotions function: they are 360° feedback loops. By that I mean they are an urge to perform an action that negates the urge. Take hunger as an example. Hunger drives eating that in turn makes hunger go away, so this is a 360° feedback loop. Another example is pity. This emotion drives the action of helping someone in difficulty, and once you have helped them, they are no longer in difficulty; so the emotion of pity switches off. Similarly, biological humiliation is driven by an attack on biological fitness. This drives a revenge response that is a reprisal attack on the source of the humiliation. If this is successful, it neutralises the threat and negates the humiliation. Evolutionary theory would agree that revenge is indeed sweet!

In the model described in the diagram (Figure 4), the combination of affectation and suppression means that the action necessary to make the original urge go away does not occur. We can therefore conclude that the urge remains and becomes a permanent urge. This permanence is the origin of compulsion in certain psychiatric disorders. The misidentification of the urge results in an action that does not make the urge go away, so the feedback loop is broken. We can illustrate this using a thermostat as an example. A biological emotion and a thermostat both work the same way: a set of circumstances triggers an action that negates the original circumstance. In the case of the thermostat in your heating system, a set of circumstances—the house is too cold—causes an action routine: the boiler is switched on. This defeats the circumstances that originally caused the action routine; so when it is no longer too cold, the thermostat cuts out and the boiler switches off. Now imagine that a thermostat in your living room controls the heating system for the whole house. If you turn off the radiators in your living room, then when the thermostat turns on the boiler, it will heat the whole house except the room where the thermostat is situated; so there is no mechanism to turn the heating system off, and the living room will stay cold and the rest of the house will get warmer and warmer. We could say that the heating system is compulsively on, since the mechanism to turn it on works fine, but the one to turn it off has been disengaged. The boiler will remain permanently on until summer arrives.

We can now perform an analysis of how a person whose emotional behaviour had become muddled in this way would form concepts of emotion, and how this would affect how he or she acts in the light of the 2x2 matrices (Tables 2 and 3) of the aforementioned chapter (Section A: Foundations – The Theoretical Starting Point). We have to first consider each emotion in isolation, and secondly, we have to consider the impact of the crossing-over problem. The situation looks like this:

With respect to emotion 4 (in isolation), the individual is suppressing the behaviour (this is the top right-hand quadrant of Tables 2 and 3 in the chapter The Theoretical Starting Point if you need to refer back). We would, therefore, expect them to be able to correctly recognise that emotion in other people, but be completely unaware that it arises in themselves. Emotion 4 is a product of evolution by natural selection and is supposed to drive an action that increases their biological fitness. However, clearly this process has been disrupted in our subject. This is a human, and unlike other species, they can form concepts of future emotion. Rather than the emotion driving the action, they calculate actions that will strategise emotional outcomes, so the causality of this process has been reversed: they are trying to goal-seek emotional outcomes. To optimise their biological fitness, they should be calculating the action that emotion 4 is supposed to drive, but they do not acknowledge that they experience emotion 4 because they do not demonstrate the behaviour.

With respect to emotion 7, they are affecting the behaviour (i.e. the top left-hand quadrant of Tables 2 and 3). They therefore have an incorrect belief that they can identify emotion 7 in themselves, and will continue to pursue a course of action without being able to determine when a satisfactory outcome is achieved.

Now let's build in the impact of the crossing-over problem:

Normally with behaviour affected by an individual, that person comes to see the stimulus for the affectation to be the cause of the emotion—they have a false understanding of its cause. However, in this situation, the Affectation Stimulus for the behaviour of emotion 7 is the Biological Stimulus for emotion 4, and since emotion 4 never drives the action that would negate it, the stimulus is permanent. Therefore, the behaviour associated with emotion 7 is controlled by a switch that can turn on, but cannot turn off. They will therefore perceive themselves as permanently experiencing emotion 7—they will have a perpetual urge leading to a compulsive action. It will not be possible for them to realise that their sense of emotion 7 is actually caused by emotion 4's Biological Stimulus, because they have no sense that they are experiencing emotion 4—they simply are unable to acknowledge it. It would be all too easy to conclude that emotion 4 simply drives the action of emotion 7, but this is a human, and they are goal-seeking emotional outcomes based on a concept of an emotion that has a double misconception in it: identity and causality. Because the cause of emotion 4 just keeps on pumping, the behaviour of emotion 7 will be permanently on display. They consider themselves to be permanently suffering from the problem that emotion 7 is supposed to rectify, and their attempts to rectify this problem are compulsive and never-ending. And as a result, they are stuck in a loop.

There is a side issue here, that appears to be a problem at first glance but on reflection, turns out to be a red herring: with respect to emotion 7 (as properly caused), they appear to be suppressing the behaviour. However, they are persistently and compulsively performing an action whose biological intent is to negate the Biological Stimulus of emotion 7, so emotion 7, in a biological sense, would almost certainly never arise. So this situation causes a bizarre human contradiction: they would never experience emotion 7 despite thinking that they are experiencing it as a permanent state. This is a radical and persistent contradiction that is the root of their compulsion.

A person in this situation of emotional crossing over will compulsively perform an action that is inappropriate to the circumstances that they face. Observed from the outside, this person would almost certainly be judged to have obsessive-compulsive symptoms. But the hypothetical structure that we have described is entirely rational, so we now have the beginning of a scientific hypothesis that compulsiveness is logical.

There are two important questions that this hypothetical analysis suggests: the first is, how could a person get in such a tangle in the first place? and the second is, how is it possible to break such a person out of it? I suspect that both questions may prove quite hard to answer. To the first, I have been trying to explain that we are all exposed to layers of tactically deceptive behaviour and that it is not that hard to arrive at a misidentification of one of our own emotional states. Once we have made the incorrect identification, then it is very difficult to rectify. The crossing-over problem that I am describing here could result from a person being exposed to multiple distortions at the same time. To answer the second question, you have to consider what you would see if you were this person's therapist: you would see a compulsive action that is inappropriate for that person's circumstances, but you cannot see the emotions that drive them. If you ask the person what drives them, you are asking them to talk about emotions of which they have no concept of experiencing. However, we know which emotional behaviour they are affecting: it is the one that is the Biological Stimulus for the action that is compulsively performed (emotion 7). So, we could start by training them to cease affecting it, which will seem like suppressing it in the first instance. But we are suppressing an emotional behaviour that we are habitually affecting, or trying to break that habit. It is only when we have broken that habit that it will be possible to determine which emotional behaviour was being suppressed (emotion 4). Once the effect of affecting emotion 7 has been eliminated, we can then consider which emotion does not seem to be responding to normal stimuli (namely, emotion 4).

In *The Logic of Self-Destruction* I built the theory using thought experiments that used real emotions as their raw material. I could do this because everybody lives in a world where tactical deception of emotional behaviour is commonplace and therefore this is easy to relate to as a normal human. It helps to have a real example.

However, here we are building a theory using thought experiments that employ compound emotional misconceptions. This is something that normal people may not experience, and people with psychiatric conditions may not understand that they are actually experiencing, so we have a need to analyse this in a more mathematical or diagrammatical way.

Now that we have completed the analysis, we can tentatively replace the numbered emotions with named ones. The purpose of this is to take a dry mathematical formulation of the problem and attempt to put a human face on it. We could recreate the emotional diagram used above (Figure 4) like so (Figure 5):

FIGURE 5: SWITCHED BEHAVIOUR IN SPECIFIC EMOTIONS

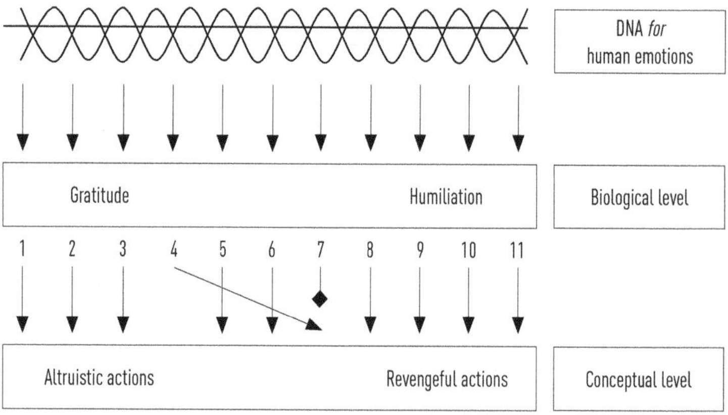

I have included on the scale, two approximately opposing biological emotions (gratitude and humiliation) together with the two actions (altruistic and revengeful) they would drive assuming they are not messed around by tactical deception. I picked these two biological emotions by way of example; I could have chosen many other pairs. I have now constructed a hypothetical individual who is compulsively revengeful in certain situations where they should cooperate. I have constructed a hypothetical model of a human who behaves in a compulsively self-destructive manner—a person who certainly has severe problems of a sort that a psychiatrist would describe as obsessive-compulsive—and this model requires them to have nothing wrong with their genetic make-up or their brain functionality.

Mathematics is a technique for solving real-world empirical problems. I can work out that two apples plus two apples equals four apples by mental imagining; but when I try to imagine six piles of five apples, my imagination gets clogged up with apples. By removing apples from the process, I unclog my imagination and give it scope to solve bigger problems. Mathematics is the process of looking at real-world problems and then freeing the imagination by eliminating the world. John von Neumann is one of the few mathematicians to accept that they probably never thought of a problem to solve that did not start with an empirical observation. As he observed, 'it is very hard for any mathematician to believe that mathematics is a purely empirical science or that all mathematical ideas originate in empirical subjects.'[81]

The four basic modes of corruption to our concepts of emotion (described in Table 2), and the corresponding four basic modes of deriving a self-destructive action from a corrupt concept of emotion (described in Table 3), give us a theoretical framework. We can understand how a biological emotion that drives a survival-enhancing action is transformed into a distorted concept of emotion by tactical deception of the emotional behaviour; and from here we rationally derive a self-destructive action. If I do this with only one element of behavioural distortion, I can construct this in my imagination, and leaving humanity in there does not unduly clog up my imagination. When I try to multiply the problem—consider two or more tactical deceptions occurring in two or more emotions simultaneously—then my imagination gets clogged up with humanity. I have to convert the whole process into a form of mathematics. Once I have done this, my imagination is free to run riot, and I decided to simply mash it all up. What I discovered is that by doing this I could *invent* a mental illness. Note the emphasis! I am not claiming that I have *discovered* a mental illness, or *described* an actual mental illness in a real human being. What I am doing is demonstrating that if we hybridise misconceptions of emotion in this particular way, then compulsive action is a rationally derived outcome.

This, of course, only half achieves the objective. In a results-oriented world, people are not interested in hearing about problems; they want solutions. But with a problem like mental illness that causes untold misery for sufferers and their families, and costs governments billions of dollars in lost productivity, criminal damage, treatment and internment, we are facing a huge problem that we cannot even define. If I can just define the problem, then I hope that this is a sufficiently valuable contribution. At this stage, I have not addressed how the person's behaviour in our case study became so distorted in the first place. But we know that some people compulsively repeat actions that do not serve their apparent interests, for example, by compulsively washing their hands, and it would appear that such people are trapped in a feedback loop. What I have tried to demonstrate is how this could be rational. By turning concepts of emotion into a mathematical structure, we can turn psychiatry into a branch of logic.

ACTION DRIVERS AND ACTION INHIBITORS

So far, we have considered emotions that are action drivers. The problem with such decent, simple ideas is that, generally, it is not long before they turn into messy, complicated ones. Anger, humiliation and pity are examples of emotions that are action drivers. The slightly broad way that I characterise emotions also clearly includes hunger and thirst as action drivers, but I do not explore these much because normal people (i.e. ones without a psychiatric diagnosis attached to their name) tend not to perform tactical deception with the associated behaviour.

However, I also need to acknowledge that some emotions, for example shame, are action inhibitors. Looking at the broader characterisation of emotions, we could also include tiredness as an action inhibitor. There are some strange action inhibitors that we do not normally think of as emotions. For example, there are biological inhibitors that stop you having sex with your close family members, or eating other humans. Under normal circumstances, these inhibitors never switch off; so, paradoxically, we have almost no awareness of them ever being switched on. We cannot deny that incest and cannibalism occur in humans, but biologically speaking this is anomalous. I will explore biologically anomalous sex acts later in this book (Compulsion in Human Sexuality) and attempt to explain why the majority of human sexual activity cannot be explained by biology. Biological inhibitors that never switch off, such as those that prevent cannibalism and incest, are usually referred to as 'taboos'. But so nebulous is our conception of such important biological inhibitors, that in normal parlance we do not even have a name for them.

There are other inhibiting emotions if we look elsewhere in the animal kingdom. Many prey species will freeze when they see a predator before the predator sees them. This freeze response is driven by an inhibiting emotion. It seems reasonable to assume that we have inherited this response from our ancestors, who roamed the plains, but humans no longer have predators and so this response is something that most humans will not experience. But the expression 'she froze in fear' is a staple cliché of somewhat unimaginative fiction writing in the thriller genre.

There are some complications with trying to distinguish between driving and inhibiting emotions in the real world. For example, people often talk of guilt and shame as if they are synonymous, but I use these words very differently. Guilt is a driving emotion that causes you to perform onerous social obligations—like calling up your aged auntie on her birthday; but shame is an inhibitor that stops you performing antisocial actions—like stealing old ladies' handbags. Here I am trying to restrict the meanings of the words to avoid confusion. Another slight complication is that some emotions can be either drivers or inhibitors depending upon the circumstances. For example, hunger is usually considered to be a driver, since it causes the action of seeking food. But people who experience the extremes of hunger during famines or while imprisoned in concentration camps, start to become more obsessed with conserving energy than seeking food—at which point, hunger has inverted and become an inhibiting emotion. However, I do not want us to get distracted by these ideas at the moment. Each of the great works in the tradition of British Empiricism (Hobbes' *Leviathan*, Locke's *An Essay Concerning Human Understanding*, Hume's *A Treatise of Human Nature*, etc.) contains a lengthy discourse of at least two chapters describing each emotion: what it does and what its purpose is. I want to avoid repeating this here; so I am mostly going to talk in the abstract about driving emotions and inhibiting emotions. That way, we can consider their interaction without getting lost in obscure biology or human functionality. Since we are talking about how humans can become confused about their emotions, we also avoid getting lost in my confusions or your confusions.

If tactical deception with emotional behaviour causes us to form false concepts of the emotion, then, firstly, does this work the same way with driving and inhibiting emotions? Secondly, does a human deduce a self-destructive action from a false concept of an emotion in the same way in each case?

Let us start by considering the derivation of the understanding of the emotion from behaviour that has been modified by tactical deception. An emotion is a function that converts a set of circumstances into an action state. Pity converts the circumstance of seeing someone in difficulty into the action state of offering assistance. Shame converts the circumstance of seeing an old lady on a dark and lonely backstreet into the *non*-action state of *not* mugging her. Without the state of shame, hunger and other emotional drivers would convert this situation into the action state of stealing her handbag. We often underestimate how important shame is in our daily lives. In almost every social situation, there is an obnoxious action available to us that can benefit us at someone else's expense, and yet, without thinking, we usually choose not to do it.

As with driving emotions, inhibiting emotions also form 360° feedback loops. The thought of mugging the old lady causes shame, which inhibits the act of mugging her. The fact that I did not mug her causes the feeling of shame to go away. An inhibiting emotion causes a state of non-action that negates the inhibition. That last sentence is perhaps the only legitimate one I have ever written that contains a quadruple negative.

It is important to note that the emotion is the function and not the action state. As described before, a concept of an emotion is a derivative of behaviour. This is the case irrespective of what the action state is. If the behaviour is suppressed, we disrupt the ability to identify the emotion, and this is the same whether the emotion is intended to drive or inhibit an action (Table 2). Similarly, if the behaviour is affected, we deduce false causes of the emotion. The word for an emotion, therefore (strictly speaking), references whatever is the cause of the behaviour. We generally presume this to be a feeling that underlies the emotion itself, but when the behaviour has been modified by a tactical deception, this presumption is no longer correct.

How then does this impact action? The first thing to realise is that with emotions that inhibit action, the goal is to avoid the emotion by not performing an action. If we are trying to compute an action that achieves an emotional goal, then if the emotion of shame causes us *not* to act, then it is difficult to understand why we would seek to compute a non-action to achieve the non-state of shame. The emotional goal is the avoidance of shame and tiredness. If we try to achieve this with an incorrect concept of these emotions, what would be the rational consequence?

With emotions that drive actions, the origin of the self-destructive action is that humans reverse the causality: in animals the emotion pushes the action, and in humans the action pulls the emotion. We compute the action that would give rise to a future emotional state, and if we have an incorrect idea of that emotion, we deduce an action that damages us. With emotions that inhibit actions, I cannot see why a human would reverse the causality in this way. The computation of a non-action that would achieve the future non-state of shame is the same non-action that achieves the current non-state of shame. (Aha! Is that a quadruple negative or a pair of double negatives?) I can only avoid an action that would avoid my current shame and, since we are only looking at the present tense here, this is the same thing as my current shame inhibiting me performing the action.

In other words, unlike actions that drive emotions, reversing the causality does not alter the outcome. This is rather like the arithmetic we learned when we were seven years old: $x + y$ is the same as $y + x$, but $x - y$ is not the same as $y - x$. With inhibiting emotions, our ability to understand the emotion in the future does not alter its operation even when we have a misconception of it. This makes emotions that inhibit actions much easier to understand. If I suppress the emotion of shame, then it simply stops the inhibition, and this is not complicated. Endurance athletes suppress the emotion of tiredness, and so they keep running, but this only happens in the present tense. Every endurance athlete knows that at some point in the future, they will be unable to suppress their tiredness anymore.

When inhibiting emotions are suppressed by a third party, it simply elevates the lack of inhibition to a mass phenomenon. Genocide involves the collective suppression of shame, and this eliminates the idea that killing people en masse is wrong. We could update Table 3 for the effect on the action where the concept of an inhibiting emotion is corrupt, but it is so straightforward (Table 4) that (hopefully) this is not difficult to understand:

TABLE 4: EFFECT ON HUMAN ACTION WHEN INHIBITING EMOTIONS ARE
HABITUALLY CORRUPTED

Effect on the action	Affect	Suppress	
First person	Your action is inhibited in circumstances that other people would consider odd. (For example, a nun feels shame over lewd thoughts.)	Your action is not inhibited in a way that other people would consider normal. (For example, a pickpocket suppresses shame when stealing.)	The inhibition does not work in accordance with instinctive biological emotions.
Second/third person	Public morality demands that an action that would otherwise appear natural is inhibited. (For example, in many countries, it is illegal to urinate in public.)	A previously inhibited action becomes generally accepted. (For example, we expand sexual tolerance to include sex acts previously considered perverted.)	Public morality parts company with biological emotion as a regulator of human action.
	Repressive.	Permissive.	

Relative to the logical complexities of being confused about emotions that drive actions, this is straightforward by comparison. However, the suppression of emotional behaviour results in our having an impaired ability to identify our own emotions. In *Part I: The Human Algorithm* of *The Logic of Self-Destruction*, I pointed out that when we are confused about the identity of our own emotion, we do not necessarily have to mistakenly identify our own emotion as another. We could identify it as something else altogether.[82]

What I want to consider now is, what happens if we mistake an emotion that drives an action for one that inhibits an action? When we have answered this question, we can then examine what happens when this happens the other way round.

THE ANTI-COMPULSION

In the first chapter in this section: A Compulsion to Perform an Action, the reasoning behind the compulsion to act inappropriately involved a mix-up between emotional action drivers. Continuing with the same method of reasoning, let us take the following (Figure 6) to be a model of a very simple human who has got only two emotions, but has still managed to get them into a tangle:

FIGURE 6: A MODEL OF AN ANTI-COMPULSION

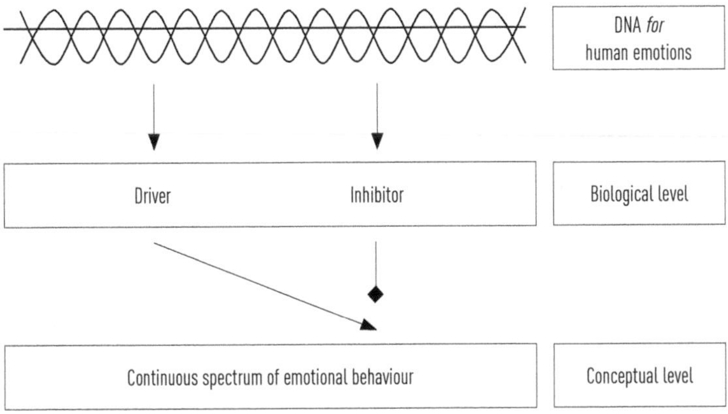

		DNA *for* human emotions
Driver	Inhibitor	Biological level
Continuous spectrum of emotional behaviour		Conceptual level

This person has one biological emotion that drives action and another that inhibits action, and by a compound manipulation of the behaviour, they have found themselves in the situation where the Biological Stimulus for the driving emotion has become the Affectation Stimulus for the inhibiting emotion; so only the behaviour for the inhibiting emotion is displayed. We can repeat the analysis that we performed in the aforementioned chapter and consider first the two emotions separately, and then look at the inter-causality that relates to the crossing over.

With respect to the inhibiting emotion, our hypothetical individual is affecting the inhibiting emotional behaviour, and so has an incorrect belief that they are identifying the inhibiting emotion in themselves. This simply acts as a constraint on action, because with inhibiting emotions we do not get the inversion of causality that arises with driving emotions.

As in the previous case, with respect to the driving emotion (in isolation), they suppress the behaviour and are therefore able to recognise that emotion in other people, but remain unaware that they are experiencing it themselves. The biological emotion is supposed to drive an action, but is not doing so in this case. Clearly, this situation is self-destructive in isolation: they think they are experiencing an emotion that inhibits action. Therefore, trying to compute an action that achieves a future emotional goal is irrelevant in this case. To optimise their biological fitness, they should be calculating the action that the driving emotion is supposed to drive. However, they do not acknowledge that they experience it because they do not demonstrate the behaviour.

Let us consider the impact of the crossing-over.

Driving emotions are feedback mechanisms. They arise because the human (or animal) needs to rectify something, and the stronger the need to rectify, the stronger the emotional urge. A human, at any point in time, will have multiple emotions, and the one that is strongest will tend to become dominant over the others and drive the action that occurs next. If you are both hungry and thirsty, then the stronger emotion will determine whether you drink or eat first. This action cancels out the urge to act. Here, the driving emotion is an Affectation Stimulus for an inhibitor; so the action does not occur and the feedback mechanism is broken. Failure to act on the driving emotion results in it becoming steadily stronger, leading the inhibition to become all-embracing and eventually consume the individual. The inhibition will become this individual's dominant emotion on an almost permanent basis. The negative feedback mechanism has turned into a positive feedback mechanism, where the urge to not act keeps getting stronger. This is a compulsion to *not* do something that biology dictates you should do—what I generically call an 'Anti-Compulsion'.

This is so much mathematical theory, but what we are really interested in are human problems. We need to translate this mathematical theory back into the human world and consider whether we have explained anything of value. What we need is a situation where someone has an urge to perform an action, but a reason not to do it. We also need this situation to continue over a long period of time. The psychiatric casebooks are positively overflowing with examples.

If a person is under pressure to diet (say because they are an actor or dancer) and this situation continues over a long period, then it is quite possible that an individual will affect shame as a strategy to counteract their urge to eat. This situation repeats until it becomes a conditioned reflex. This model is based entirely upon the assumption of a rational agent responding to their concepts of emotional drivers and inhibitors. The Biological Stimulus for a driver (hunger) becomes an Affectation Stimulus for an inhibitor (shame). Here, we have constructed a simple model for what psychiatrists call 'anorexia nervosa'. I would call this an 'Anti-Compulsion with respect to eating'—a name that is precisely descriptive of the situation. Anorexia nervosa is usually considered to be an 'eating disorder', but psychiatry, without a theory of causality, can only describe such things by reference to their symptoms. Searching the academic press regarding theories for its causes turns up little beyond vague hypotheses. However, here we have a concise hypothesis that is laid out causally and assumes that the agent is a logical computational device, goal-seeking their emotional outcomes.

The experience of World War I also provides us with many clear examples of Anti-Compulsions. World War I was perhaps a turning point in the development of psychiatry, because the psychological casualties exceeded the physical ones. This was quite different to all previous wars, and psychiatrists suddenly had to cope with psychological symptoms that they had never seen before. Men dug themselves into trenches and bombarded each other with heavy artillery continuously for months on end. The obvious urge is to run away or to cry out in fear, but this is prohibited. An additional natural response to this circumstance is involuntary urination or defecation, and these urges are suppressed over long periods. It is entirely to be expected that, eventually, soldiers will seek to manage their urge to do these things by affecting shame—an inhibiting emotion. Mutism was very common in traumatised soldiers—what I would call an Anti-Compulsion with reference to talking. Another example was an inability to walk, including the display of extraordinary gaits—an Anti-Compulsion with respect to walking.[83] More bizarrely, soldiers occasionally displayed Anti-Compulsions with respect to defecation or urination that eventually caused the body to bloat to a grotesque and agonising degree. It is easy to visualise that an Anti-Compulsion with reference to urination gives rise to much more serious medical complications than an Anti-Compulsion with reference to eating, and such people can experience terrible deaths in a few days without medical intervention. The model of Anti-Compulsion that we have constructed makes these symptoms seem almost obvious—even predictable.

There was one, almost universal, symptom shared by World War I soldiers with various forms of Anti-Compulsion, and that was acute sexual dysfunction. This does not fit so easily into the model described here. But at the time, in a relatively oppressive Edwardian society, shame was most commonly associated with the inhibition of sex. Now, the perception of shame (which is, of course, a mistaken perception, since it is habitually affected) is a near permanent state. As with anorexia nervosa, the psychiatric profession has made little progress in understanding these symptoms. In World War I, they were collectively called 'shell shock'—an expression originally coined by soldiers themselves. This term was initially adopted by the medical profession, simply because they did not have a word of their own. Now, the medical profession has renamed this as 'post-traumatic stress disorder', but renaming it with a more formal, technical expression does nothing to explain its cause.

Science is generally concerned with understanding the relation-ship between causes and effects. In medical terms, we would talk about the aetiology of a disease and its symptoms. In the case of mental illness, it is often easy to get causes and effects confused. For example, the psychiatric literature often states that a symptom of anorexia nervosa is 'low self-esteem'. The model that we have cre-ated involves the affectation of an inhibiting emotion that ultimately becomes to be displayed almost permanently. This could be any inhibiting emotion, but is likely to be shame. A permanent belief in shame is *not* a symptom of the condition. It *is* the mechanism; so we need to make a distinction: 'low self-esteem' is a myth that psychia-trists have about their patients, whereas the permanent perception of shame is a myth that the patient has about him or herself. 'Low self-esteem' is not a symptom; it is a form of self-perception that comes about through systematic affectation of the behaviour of shame.

Once we recognise that all the Anti-Compulsions in the psychi-atric casebook should be grouped together, we can start to cast the net wider. We can find in the psychiatric case histories an exam-ple of an Anti-Compulsion with respect to virtually every human function. Shyness is an Anti-Compulsion with respect to social situ-ations. As already mentioned, Hippocrates first described shyness in 400 BC, but the early editions of the DSM did not consider it a psy-chiatric disorder. Without a theory of causality, there is a natural tendency to regard situations according to how serious their conse-quences are—Anti-Compulsions with respect to social situations are not life-threatening like Anti-Compulsions with respect to eating, but the theory described here suggests that they have the same causal mechanism. The APA appeared to recognise this in DSM–III, where they officially classified shyness as a mental disorder calling it 'social anxiety disorder'.

At the other end of the spectrum, I can think of no reason why it is not possible to have an Anti-Compulsion with respect to breathing. However, I doubt you will find this in the psychiatric casebook. When it happens, you first try the Heimlich manoeuvre, and then you check to see if they have swallowed their tongue, but a person in this condition will likely be dead before anybody thinks to call a psychiatrist. The cause of death will be described as a 'seizure', which is a catch-all term for medically unexplained, sudden death.

THE LIBERTINE COMPULSION

As explained in the previous chapter in this section, an Anti-Compulsion involves the substitution of an emotional driver with an emotional inhibitor. Let us now consider the substitution the other way round (Figure 7). Once again, this is a mathematical model of a stripped-down human who only has two emotions that have become muddled:

FIGURE 7: A MODEL OF A LIBERTINE COMPULSION

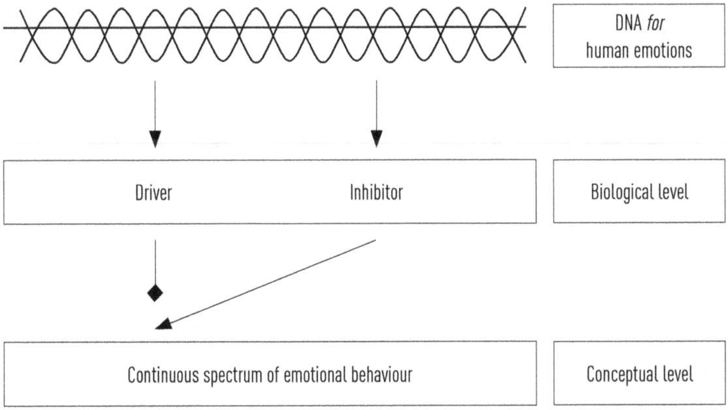

	DNA *for* human emotions
Driver	Inhibitor	Biological level
Continuous spectrum of emotional behaviour	Conceptual level

Like our previous hypothetical person, this one has an emotion that drives action and another that inhibits action. The trigger for the inhibiting emotion causes the behaviour for the driving emotion to be displayed.

In the same way that the third Harry Potter book no longer

needed to explain the rules of quidditch, we can get straight to the point. With respect to the inhibiting emotion, our hypothetical individual is failing to display the corresponding behaviour. He has no concept that he experiences this emotion, and so has switched off the inhibiting effect. This is not complicated since we do not need to worry about any inversion of causality.

With respect to the driving emotion, he is affecting the behaviour, and therefore, he has an incorrect belief that he experiences that emotion. He thinks that he understands what causes it, but what actually causes it are the circumstances that would normally cause the inhibiting emotion. A person who affects an emotion would normally keep repeating an action without being able to understand whether they achieve the emotional goal that they seek. However, in this case before we can jump to that conclusion, we need to consider the interdependence of the two emotions—what I previously called the crossing-over problem.

This hypothetical human is seeking an emotional outcome that is caused by performing an act that would be inhibited in a normal person. The point of inhibiting emotions is to stop you performing asocial or antisocial actions. It is therefore completely rational that this person will compulsively perform asocial or antisocial actions. They are doing this because they believe it achieves an emotional outcome, without being able to determine whether they were successful in achieving that outcome. However, they have attained a state where they regard an inhibiting emotion—such as shame—as an emotional goal to be achieved. They compulsively perform an action that is abhorrent to society without actually achieving any emotional fulfilment.

The term 'libertine' means a person who performs an action considered contrary to public morality. In an increasingly liberal world, the word has fallen into disuse, and I rather like bringing archaic words back into use. You can use them without needing to change their sense—rather like finding a really useful tool in your grandfather's garden shed. If we look at the historic use of this word, it has shifted as public morality shifted. In the seventeenth century, it could be applied to someone who danced too much, or to a woman who refused to do her husband's laundry. At the time, that could be enough for you to be committed to an asylum for the insane. This, of course, was seen as being for your benefit: to inculcate in you an appropriate decorum considered acceptable to the morality of the age.

By the late eighteenth century, the word applied more to a freethinker, which at that time could include someone who was suspected of being an atheist. By the twentieth century, the word was almost eliminated from current use. The expression 'Libertine Compulsion' is intended to describe a condition of being compelled to perform socially abhorrent actions.

In the human world, we can find many examples. The most obvious is a serial killer. It would appear that many of them seek to obtain fulfilment from an action that causes their own shame. However, they have no ability to determine whether performing the act of killing actually brings about the fulfilment or not. Killing, being an antisocial act, actually does cause shame, but they have no awareness of this because they do not display the behaviour. They are therefore trapped in a feedback loop: increased shame creates an even greater urge to perform the action again.

Anecdotal evidence would appear to show that for many infamous serial killers, as they developed, their killing became more extreme and more audacious, until the police were often heard to say that it appeared they actually wanted to be caught. This is precisely what this model would predict, since shame needs an audience to become complete. If the shame is actually the emotional goal, then becoming more gruesome generates more of it. Accelerating brutality is therefore entirely rational given the combination of drivers and inhibitors, and how this rational agent would interpret them.

Let us return to the thermostat metaphor. A set of circumstances (being too cold or too hot) switches on a mechanism (the heating system or air conditioning system) that eventually causes the set of circumstances to be undone. At this point, the switch is turned off. The thermostat on your heating system and air conditioning system operate in opposite directions—one switches on when it is too cold and the other switches on when it is too hot. If you are careless, you can set the thermostat on your heating system at a lower temperature than that on your air conditioning system. In this circumstance, it is certain that it will be either cold enough to switch on the heating—in which case it will become hot enough to switch on the air conditioning; or it will be hot enough to switch on the air conditioning—in which case it will become cold enough to switch on the heating. Either way, both systems will eventually be switched on simultaneously. The two systems constantly defeat one another in a feedback loop that is a contradiction of mechanical systems. It does not mean that there is anything wrong with your heating or air conditioning systems, other than the thermostats being set at the wrong level. To complete the analogy, we could say that a serial killer's compulsion to bring about his own shame comes about because he has two thermostats operating in opposite directions—one drives and the other inhibits. The situation he finds himself in is, of course, a form of contradiction. But one that is entirely rational in a person whose thermostats have become set in a conflicting pattern.

Are there other examples of Libertine Compulsions in humans? Alcoholism may be one. My anecdotal evidence is that shame is a major component of alcoholism, which is why they so often drink in secret and resist admitting their problem. One friend of mine with a serious alcohol problem would leave her phone, purse and coat in a sequence of bars, and the next day would be too ashamed to recover them, so I would do this for her. A bar would seem, to most of us, to be the last place where you would be ashamed to be drunk, but the model of compulsion that we have constructed here involves the confusion between driving and inhibiting emotions. It is possible that the next day she thinks she is ashamed, but is actually incorrectly identifying that emotion in herself. However, alcoholism is a good example of a compulsion where it is difficult to know whether it is a Libertine Compulsion or a regular compulsion, and it may be that there are different forms of it that fit each model separately.

Another possible example of a Libertine Compulsion is child molesting; so this is a good moment to take a detour and discuss how compulsion interacts with biology to create that strange human phenomenon that we call 'sexuality'.

COMPULSION IN HUMAN SEXUALITY

The only form of sex that could be considered purely biological is copulation between a male and a female when the female is in oestrus. We explain our urge to perform sex that results in procreation with evolutionary biology. In humans, non-procreative sex acts cannot be explained this way. What I am attempting to construct here in Section B: Compulsions is a theoretical map of all the forms of compulsion observed in humans. I now want to explore whether we should consider non-procreative sex acts to be forms of non-biological compulsion.

The list is pretty extensive: masturbation, foot fetishism, homosexuality, paedophilia, anal sex, oral sex, etc. If we look at the history of psychiatry, the performance of every one of these sex acts has been considered to be a form of madness. Throughout the eighteenth and nineteenth centuries, there was confusion as to whether masturbation was a cause of madness or a form of madness in its own right. This view survived until Freud. Similarly, almost all the literature before Freud considered 'nymphomania' to be a form of madness. Women were often interned in asylums for a single act of fornication. If your wife was unfaithful, then this was a simpler way of ridding yourself of her than the divorce courts. For instance, Donatien Alphonse François, Marquis de Sade ran away with his teenage sister-in-law and had a scandalous affair. This behaviour was considered so depraved that it was completely off the scale of the contemporary moral spectrum. The stunt earned him his own personal psychiatric diagnosis: 'libertine dementia'.[84]

It is easy to dismiss this as the ignorance of a prior age, but homosexuality was also considered to be a form of mental illness in comparatively recent times. The APA declared it to be a 'sociopathic personality disturbance' in 1952. But then, in the 1974 seventh printing of DSM-II, they changed their mind and removed it entirely. The original opinion has almost certainly not been completely dispelled. This shift largely resulted from the research of Evelyn Hooker. In 1957, she completely turned medical opinion on its head by demonstrating that open and consensual homosexuals were as happy and well-adjusted as heterosexual couples.[85] The elimination of homosexuality from DSM was also partly due to lobbying by the gay community. Normally, we would not consider the opinions of non-scientists to be a valid reason for shifting scientific judgement, and the susceptibility of the psychiatric profession on this demonstrates how weak their science is.

The view that non-procreative sex acts are normal has been reinforced by the successive discoveries of such acts in the animal kingdom. For example, a recent discovery is that prostitution occurs in the animal kingdom.[86] The most bizarre animals that have been observed performing this behaviour are penguins; a full discussion of the barter-value of regurgitated fish is beyond the scope of this book, however. We have known for some time that lesbianism is common in seagulls, which completely baffles evolutionary theorists because it is a form of sexual practice that is completely antithetical to what evolutionary theory tells us should be the goal of a living organism. However, lesbian seagulls often raise a chick due to normal sexual activity by one of them; so this is not true lesbianism, but two females cooperating in the raising of a family. The female that is not the biological mother is just a victim of brood parasitism—a common problem in the bird world. Bonobos, who are genetically the closest relatives to humans, engage in a whole range of sex acts common in humans, including homosexuality, mutual masturbation, kissing and oral sex.[87] These discoveries in the animal kingdom make human sexuality seem closer to biology, but there is a widespread tendency to over-extrapolate these observations. For example, there are approximately 400 species where

homosexual acts have been observed, but lifelong homosexual preference is very rare. Other than humans, about the only other animal
that demonstrates lifelong homosexual preference is domestic sheep,
with the bighorn sheep being one of the only wild animals.[88] Bonobos that engage in occasional homosexual sex acts still perform
heterosexual sex, and therefore breed normally. The usual evolutionary explanation of this is that they use mutual sexual gratification
as a form of social bonding and a way of reconciling social conflict,
and this enhances survival. But this argument is quite difficult to
fully state in terms of how it works at a gene level.

Despite occasional excitement in the media about the discovery
of a 'gay gene', the evolutionary origins of homosexuality continue
to mystify. The only explanation that I consider credible is the 'kin
selection hypothesis'.[89] This argues that it is empirically demonstrable that with the birth of each successive son to a woman, the
probability of that son being homosexual increases by about 33 per
cent.[90] It is thought that this occurs not for genetic reasons, but
because the mother develops an immune response to certain male
antigens to which she is exposed during pregnancy with a boy. This
impacts upon male brain development to an increasing degree with
each such pregnancy.[91] The reason that this immune reaction is not
eliminated by natural selection is that it mainly arises in large families, which have a disproportionately high chance of having at least
one gay son. Having a spare male in a large family—the beneficial
uncle—increases the chances of the nieces and nephews surviving
and thriving, so the gene for the immune reaction propagates. This
argument supports the idea that homosexuality is an orientation and
not a choice, but since it is not genetically heritable there is no gene
for homosexuality as such. I find this hypothesis compelling,
although empirical studies are inconclusive that this actually
occurs.[92] There are three other weaknesses with this argument: it
fails to translate to sheep (since gay sheep do not care for their
nieces and nephews); if it were true, we would expect lifelong
homosexual orientation to be more widespread among other species

where a single female might have successive male offspring; and lastly, it does not explain lesbianism.

De Waal, in his studies of chimpanzees, only observed a single case of forced copulation,[93] which possibly makes rape more common in humans than chimpanzees. Incest is extremely rare in advanced mammals, and evolutionary theory provides good explanations of the behavioural adaptations that avoid this. Copulation between animals that are not sexually mature is also very rare. However, if we found that rape, incest and paedophilia existed in the animal kingdom, this would not make them 'normal' in humans any more than it makes homosexuality evolutionarily explicable. We need to be careful of confusing moral judgements with scientific ones. Moral judgements are based on who—if anybody—gets harmed. This is not relevant to scientific explanation, and I would compare such a distinction to that which existed recently in psychiatry between Anti-Compulsions with respect to social situations and eating. The former was not life threatening, but the latter was; so 'social anxiety disorder' did not exist in the psychiatric lexicon, but 'anorexia nervosa' did. I am concerned with the causality of an action or orientation, without regard to whether or not someone else is harmed or considers it abhorrent. If we ignore the moral problems of whether adults consent or whether anybody gets harmed, we are left with the purely scientific problem of explaining non-procreative sex acts. My suggestion is that we should look to the mechanisms of non-biological compulsive actions principally described in the preceding four chapters here in this section.

In the early twenty-first century, we have become so sexually permissive that most forms of non-procreative sex acts have been eliminated from the DSM. The current edition DSM-V includes 'gender dysphoria' and 'ego-dystonic homosexuality'—neither of which is a diagnosis based on a sex act; rather they are based on sexual identities that are in conflict with a person's preferred identity. 'Paraphilia' (sexual arousal caused by objects or situations) and 'paedophilic disorder' are also largely diagnoses based upon an unwanted desire rather than an action.

The diagnosis of paedophilic disorder is highly suspect and is probably more of a moral judgement than a scientific one. Before we begin on this thorny subject, we need to clarify some important distinctions. Paedophilia is a sexual attraction to prepubescent children, and hebephilia to pubescent children. These are desires, whereas child molestation is an action. Generally, only the action is illegal, but in the media the terms 'paedophile' and 'child molester' are treated as having the same meaning—which they do not—and the term 'hebephile' is never used. The other important distinction concerns consent. Every country has an 'age of consent', and these vary widely across the globe from ages 12 to 21. But this does not mean that children or teenagers younger than this arbitrary age limit do not or cannot consent; rather it means that in the eyes of the law of that country, such consent is disregarded. When people disregard the fact that children do consent (and do so frequently), it blurs another distinction between consensual paedophilic or hebephilic relationships and coerced sex acts against children. The importance of this distinction concerns the question of harm. It is uncontroversial to suggest that rape of children causes huge damage, but it is less clear that damage results where children are willing participants. In most countries, many people become sexually active at an age below the age of consent. For example, almost 40 per cent of Americans lost their virginity before they were aged 16.[94] Presumably, this means that a huge percentage of the population of many countries would technically be child molesters or rapists, despite acting in ways that we should probably regard as normal for adolescents. One researcher in the field commented: 'Persuasive evidence for the harmfulness of paedophilic relationships does not yet exist, perhaps because research on childhood sexual abuse has not been sufficiently high quality to establish harm.'[95] Such a notion is truly shocking, but it often leads to arguments by experts that we should lower the age of consent in many countries.[96] Such expert views are met with prejudice. Politicians typically argue that high ages of consent protect children, but they may only protect adults from things they wish children would not do. Personally, I support an age consent of

14 or 15, since that means children of such an age can seek advice from medical professionals without legal problems arising for anyone. When considering our current prejudices, we should recall the reaction to the research of Hooker in the 1950s[97] when violent abhorrence of homosexuality was similarly pervasive. The lack of adequate research is probably due to our abhorrence of paedophilic and hebephilic relationships being so overwhelming that we cannot even contemplate funding the research.

Our understanding of paedophilia is still limited. Recent research is tending to indicate that it is a sexual orientation with respect to age, rather like homosexuality is an orientation with respect to gender. Concluding that something subject to prejudice such as paedophilia is like homosexuality, seems to undo the hard-won acceptance of the latter in society. But we must not let prejudice interfere with science. Despite these difficulties, we have established that paedophiles tend to be of below-average stature and intelligence—which indicates that it might be a problem to do with development.[98] This view is supported by the tendency for paedophiles of lower intelligence to orient towards children of a younger age. We also now know that they are usually left-handed or ambidextrous—which indicates that it might be something to do with the way the brain is wired.[99] Without any overarching theory, these correlations are little more than factoids. They might be clues, but they are not explanations. An explanation involves describing a causal structure, and evidence seems to show that it is an involuntary orientation, but our understanding of this is still poor. It was once thought that most child molesters were themselves abused in childhood, but that view has been debunked by research. I believe that the overall architecture of child molestation (as opposed to paedophilia or hebephilia) is a Libertine Compulsion. This hypothesis is supported by recent findings that not all child molesters are paedophiles—in other words, some child molesters are not sexually attracted to children.[100] But this does not help us understand paedophilia—which appears to be more of a question of brain wiring. The latter—the desire—is correlated to stature, intellect and left-handedness, and this will make child molestation more likely, but the Libertine Compulsion (which is non-biological, but still not a choice) can occur in someone without these characteristics. This would explain why some people who are not paedophilically oriented would molest children.

The sexual dysfunction of soldiers with post-traumatic stress disorder gives us some clues regarding child molestation by Catholic priests, Jewish rabbis and Imams in Muslim madrasas. The sexual urge is repressed for decades, but it is a natural urge and so it will inevitably constantly recur. In an environment where this is forbidden, it turns into shame. It is entirely predictable that eventually the yearning for sexual fulfilment (a driving emotion) and shame (an inhibiting emotion) will become entangled in a way that makes a correct identification of each emotion difficult. However, I would tend to predict that these circumstances would be more likely to lead to an Anti-Compulsion, and it is difficult to see the precise pathway that leads to a Libertine Compulsion. But, as with the most violent serial killers, many child molesters tend to demonstrate a steady increase in their deviance, which lends support to the view that an inversion has occurred where shame has become an emotional goal. What may begin as innocent play or affection will compulsively progress to whatever act would cause the greatest shame in a normal person.

This situation may arise because of the juxtaposition of a driving emotion and an inhibiting emotion, and the resultant inability to distinguish them in the correct way. Libertine Compulsions and Anti-Compulsions are a form of opposite that result from drivers being mistaken for inhibitors, or vice versa. Obviously, in the view of the Roman Catholic Church, an Anti-Compulsion with reference to sex would be a good thing (despite it being biologically dysfunctional). I would expect this condition to be quite common among priests, but obviously we do not hear anything about it because it is not morally contemptible to society and may actually be beneficial to a priest given his circumstances. Certainly, a priest in this condition is not going to be consulting a psychiatrist; so we will not read about it in the psychiatric case histories. However, if essentially the same circumstances could lead to a priest having either a Libertine Compulsion or an Anti-Compulsion, we can see this as essentially a switch that could go either way, and the direction it flips cannot reasonably be said to be within the priest's control. This makes our judgement of molesting priests purely a moral judgement based on who gets hurt and not on whether the perpetrator had a realistic choice about their compulsion. To put this in context, we need to remember that revenge and anger are biological responses to antisocial actions performed against us, and we all judge most harshly that which we most fear. This means that our judgement of Libertine Compulsions is an emotional reaction with its own evolutionary origin, but there is no evidence to support the idea of choice in the perpetrator. A parallel absurdity is the condemnation of homosexuality by religious leaders. In any case, homosexuality is just as big a problem for religious conservatives as it is for evolutionary theorists, because they cannot argue that homosexuality is contrary to 'God's will' if it occurs in bighorn sheep. Maybe if they stopped judging homosexuality, we could stop judging child molestation. Instead, we would treat it as a public health issue (rather than one for the criminal justice system), with the aim of working out a policy, based on scientific research, that results in the least harm to children, rather than rushing to judgement based upon a supposition of harm without evidence. For a start, we ought to enquire whether the harm that comes from coercing children to cooperate with a criminal prosecution exceeds that caused by consensual hebephilic relationships, which just happen to be below some arbitrary 'age of consent'. The problem here is that the legal system has no mechanism for considering whether it might be the problem rather than the solution.

If we can establish that the causality of child molestation is indeed a Libertine Compulsion, then we can start to develop new strategies for managing it. If we achieve a better understanding of the various forms of compulsion, we might be able to deprogramme

Libertine Compulsions in molesters. And since evidence supports paedophilia being an irreversible orientation, maybe we could consider intentionally programming Anti-Compulsions in paedophiles. This is of course a highly speculative idea. But currently, we have no other way of dealing with the problem other than widespread hysteria and throwing people in prison. In many countries these days, it is so easy to get your name onto a sex offenders' register that the list is too long for the police to monitor them, which results in many of the most dangerous sex offenders being unmonitored.

The lesbian, gay, bisexual and transgendered community has long-resisted comparisons with paedophilia. But we must not let prejudice interfere with science and empirical observation. To summarise, it would appear likely that both are orientations that result from development anomalies rather than genetics. They relate to preferences, rather than actions. Homosexuals have it relatively easy these days, since the associated action is no longer considered illegal or mad, if both parties are consenting adults.

Let me try to summarise from the perspective of actions. Biological sex only occurs when the female is in oestrus, and it generally occurs just enough to produce offspring. It is easy to imagine that chimpanzees are highly promiscuous, but during periods when all the females in a troupe are pregnant or nursing infants, months can go by without any sexual intercourse between adults.[101] We have known since before Darwin that heterosexual humans have sex far more than is required for the purposes of reproduction, and have sex whether or not the woman is in oestrus. If we were to perform sex purely for the purposes of fulfilling a biological function, we would do it during only one month of the year, like practically every other animal species. And who is willing to sign up for *that*? Since almost everybody at some point in their life has had a compulsion to perform sex acts that are not procreative, we now dismiss all of this as 'normal'. For someone not to have experienced this, we would probably describe him or her as asexual. In earlier periods of sexual repression, such people blended into the permanent bachelors and spinsters of the time and nobody thought anything of it. Now that people regard their sexuality as a fundamental part of their identity, asexuals have become the new abnormals. People who never experience sexual desire for either their own or the opposite sex are increasingly lobbying to be recognised as a sexual orientation. However, if we are to look at non-procreative sexual activity as some form of non-biological compulsive action, then we should probably regard asexual people as having an Anti-Compulsion with respect to sex—just a different form of non-biological compulsion to the rest of us. My suggestion is that we should not look to biology or evolutionary theory for explanations of this. Even a so-called 'healthy appetite'—which is actually biologically excessive—probably finds its best explanation in the models of compulsive action that we have built here. But which form of compulsion should we consider?

Humans are the only species that insist on having sex in secret. Shame is frequently a part of human sexuality, and contemporary liberal ideas have not really changed this. If you doubt this, consider the devastating impact of revenge-porn! This supports the idea that most human sexuality, even 'normal' sexuality, may be a product of a Libertine Compulsion.

Now we can see that we almost all 'suffer' from some form of non-biological compulsion, it places a serial killer or a child molester in a different place in the spectrum of human existence. The idea that child molesting or serial killing is a choice does not stand up to three seconds of serious consideration. Why would someone choose *that*? We have tried every conceivable way to reverse homosexuality, including electric shock therapy, brain surgery, hormones and hypnosis. Religious conservatives have even tried praying. There has not been a single instance of a scientifically peer-reviewed reversal of the condition. As a consequence, all serious-thinking people dropped the idea that being gay was a choice decades ago. Serial killing and child molesting are conditions that do not arise because of a 'moral failing', but that does not stop them being a serious challenge to society. We need to perform more research on whether willing hebephilic relationships cause lasting harm. And we need to establish a greater understanding of the makeup of molesters; and on the conditions for, and likelihood of, recidivism. Only once we have accumulated this understanding, can we devise strategies for regulation based upon the least-harm principle, bearing in mind that if the perpetrator does not have a choice, then their condition makes them a victim too. The greatest difficulty is that someone else's compulsion can make a victim of other people who did nothing other than being in the wrong place at the wrong time.

THE UNIVERSAL ANTI-COMPULSION

We are almost at the end of our mapping of the basic forms of compulsive action states in humans. If you have followed this journey from the beginning, you will have noticed that everything in this theory comes in pairs, which sometimes double up to form 2x2 matrices (four quadrants). That is indeed the case here. We have only one way left to get ourselves confused between the identities of two different emotions. However, just to be a bit tricky, our next hypothetical person has a grand total of three emotions, which is still not enough to stop them being a rather boring person to meet at a party.

We need to consider the logical outcome of a person who gets confused about the identity of two inhibiting emotions. This leads to a different form of Anti-Compulsion. I need to put the third emotion in there because a human must have a driving emotion, or it would have no reason to do anything. An inhibiting emotion without a driving emotion is an oxymoron, because what is there to inhibit if there is no drive to do anything in the first place? The third emotion is there purely to remind us of this. So let me introduce them (Figure 8). Despite the fact that their conversation is somewhat lacking in interest, they are still deserving of your compassion. Here they are:

FIGURE 8: A MODEL OF A UNIVERSAL ANTI-COMPULSION

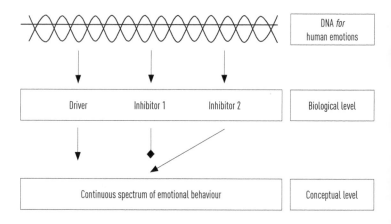

Before we can analyse this situation, we need to explore something a bit odd about inhibiting emotions. The point of an inhibiting emotion is that it stops us doing something. The phenomenon of something *not* happening does not excite our curiosity as much as something that actually does happen, and consequently, scientists do not spend a lot of time discovering the causes of non-events. It is reasonable to suppose that the emotional inhibitor that stops you having sex at funeral ceremonies is different to the emotional inhibitor that stops you eating barbecued babies. It is entirely reasonable to call these inhibitors 'emotions', since they are thermostats that convert a particular circumstance into an actions state of *not* doing something that might otherwise seem like a good idea.

However, the result of each emotional inhibitor is that we do precisely *nothing*. This alone makes it much harder for us to distinguish between inhibiting emotions, and generally, we do not even have interesting names for them. Shame is one of the only names that we have for inhibiting emotions; although as I mentioned before, some people consider guilt and shame to be synonymous. We have a name for this inhibiting emotion because we all tend to notice that it is switched on some of the time; but generally it is not, and clearly we are interested to learn the situations in which it switches on. The biological inhibitor that stops you having sex with your siblings, as mentioned earlier, is on all the time, and so we do not even notice it and do not generally have a name for it. Emotional inhibitors that never turn off—taboos—are still just emotional inhibitors like shame. Clearly, we have many inhibiting emotions because there are many circumstances when it is necessary for us to avoid a particular action. With driving emotions, these problems do not arise—few of us have difficulty understanding that hunger, pity and lust are driving mechanisms where each is triggered by a different set of circumstances, and each has an underlying biological purpose.

These complexities make it sensible to leave this situation to last. But hopefully, by this stage you are getting used to the idea of considering emotions as abstract mathematical concepts, so the fact that you probably have difficulty distinguishing your inhibiting emotions and probably do not even have distinct names for most of them will not matter as much. Strangely, this makes thinking of them in the abstract much easier, but it makes it harder to translate the results of our analysis back into human context.

So, let me explain it. For the individual introduced earlier, inhibitor 2 is supposed to stop a particular action, but clearly it is not doing so because they have suppressed the behaviour and therefore has no awareness of it. Therefore, inhibitor 2 is a thermostat that does not switch off. They believe that their inhibitor 1 is on, so they avoid the action that they believe inhibitor 1 is supposed to stop. But after they have stopped that, inhibitor 2 (which they think is inhibitor 1) is still on, so they will continue to stop doing things until they find out what will switch that inhibitor off. This is a Universal Anti-Compulsion, because it stops them doing lots of things simultaneously—possibly everything. Maybe, by chance, they might stumble upon the action that inhibitor 2 is supposed to stop. Once they stop that, inhibitor 2 switches off and they escape the Universal Anti-Compulsion. However, it is also possible that they will run out of ideas as to what actions to avoid without stumbling upon the one that will switch off inhibitor 2. In this case, they are in a permanent, inescapable state of Universal Anti-Compulsion.

The psychiatric casebook provides us with many possible examples of Universal Anti-Compulsions. The most extreme example is what a psychiatrist would call 'catalepsy', which is a total inability to move—a physical freeze-up. This can be caused by emotional triggers, such as extreme shock. Obviously, extreme danger can trigger instinctive freezing—something prey species do when they detect a predator. This is clearly an emotional inhibitor. If this situation arises often, then it becomes something you are used to and you understand what is going on. An extreme shock may give rise to an emotional inhibitor that you have never encountered before, and so how will you know what it is? The mechanism of Universal Anti-Compulsion requires a misidentification of an emotional inhibitor, so this situation is consistent with the theoretical hypothesis set out here.

An anecdotal example of catalepsy following extreme shock was the American long jumper Bob Beamon, who is said to have suffered a cataleptic seizure when told he had broken the world record by half a metre. You can find several videos of this on the internet, but it is not clear whether 'cataleptic seizure' is an accurate diagnosis of what occurred.

A more bizarre example of Universal Anti-Compulsion is 'waxy flexibility', which is a condition where a person will not move, but if you move them by forcible manipulation, they will remain in whatever position you move them to. Waxy flexibility is often associated with certain forms of schizophrenia, but, as I have said before, that is just a name for a group of symptoms. It is interesting to watch video footage of a patient suffering from waxy flexibility, and this too can easily be found on the internet.

It is conceivable that depression is a common example of Universal Anti-Compulsion, where people fall into a state of wanting to do nothing. A milder form of the same condition could be procrastination or even laziness, which arises in many of us. The cause of these latter two human phenomena is usually judged to be a moral failing, but all actions have causes, and we only make moral judgements of actions that we ourselves are not compelled to do. Psychiatrists do not consider that procrastination or laziness falls within their orbit, but neither did they think that shyness was their problem until someone decided to call it 'social anxiety disorder', thereby translating it into medicalese. The boundary between moral judgement and medical judgement is pretty hazy in this field.

However, I would like to dwell on depression because I have a personal experience with this of a highly unusual nature. People who have never suffered from depression imagine that it is something like sadness, when actually it is nothing of the kind. I once heard a psychologist refer to it as 'anger turned inward', but I disagree with that too. My experience is that it is a state where all your driving emotions flatline and an absence of drivers means you do nothing. However, thinking philosophically, it is difficult to make a distinction between all your drivers being turned off and all your inhibitors being turned on. Either way, you end up in a state where you feel that you have absolutely no reason to do anything. You do not even have a reason to escape depression, so the first lesson for anybody who has a family member with this condition is that it may be incorrect to assume that a depressed person wants the situation to change.

I suffered depression in my teens and I can honestly say that the periods of being actively depressed were not unpleasant. The problem is that, because you do nothing in that period, your life starts to fall apart and you have to deal with the consequences of this later. Also, you lose your friends. It is this cumulative effect of doing nothing for long periods of time that makes you realise that you have to escape it. But things really have to start falling apart in a major way to make you act. It is a bit like being an alcoholic, where being drunk is not the problem but dealing with the aftermath of what happened when you were drunk, is the problem. Alcoholics do not seek help until they hit rock bottom. I have always considered the period during my teens when I suffered depression as one of my most formative. You cannot understand fulfilment or contentment until you have experienced its antithesis.

So, let me now describe my unique experience with depression. When I was writing Parts I and II of *The Logic of Self-Destruction*, I built the theory around a sequence of thought experiments that I called 'Scenarios'. Each of these involved a person (or a group of people) who lived with a behavioural modification that started with a tactical deception that then became habitual. Firstly, I derived how this would alter their concept of the emotion involved, and from this I derived how it would change how they would decide to act. In this way, I could translate a corruption of innate behaviour into a form of self-destructive action.

The point of this exercise is to explain why humans are so confused about their emotions. But I am trying to explain this to people who are in turn confused about their own emotions, namely, *you*: the reader. If you live with the precise form of the behavioural manipulation that the thought experiment is trying to explore, then you would probably be unable to understand the thought experiment. This would not be due to a lack of intelligence but a problem caused by your perspective. Obviously, I also suffered from the same problems of perspective, because I too come from a family and culture where people individually and collectively manipulated their behaviour. When I was writing the book, I found that some of the Scenarios were easy to construct: I thought them up over breakfast and they were written by lunchtime. Others seemed impossible. When I was unable to write these, I started to panic: if I could not do them, then I could not finish the book. Eventually, I realised that the ones I could not do were impossible because I was trying to construct thought experiments that described my own emotional misconceptions, which is to be expected. I then went through a process of self-analysis. I deduced that I could not write a Scenario because that form of behaviour manipulation was a dominant feature of my own life, and then I searched my memory for examples of it. I could thereby work out why I could not do them, but this however, did not enable me to do them.

The eventual solution was that, through meditation, I trained myself to enter a state of depression. This caused all my own emotions to flatline so that they did not get in the way of doing the thought experiment. Obviously, in a state of depression, I had no urge to do anything, but as this state lifted I was able to complete the missing Scenarios successfully. This entire process took over a year, and there was more than one Scenario to which this process applied. I am not going to tell you which ones they were, but to this day they are the ones that I am least proud of. This could be because the circumstances under which I wrote them meant that they are not entirely freely constructed thought experiments, or it could be because my own history leaves me with the belief that that type of self-destruction is entirely normal and reasonable.

A side effect of this process is that I developed a stammer, but curiously, I only have this when I talk about my theoretical work and not when I discuss anything else. Stammering might well be a form of Anti-Compulsion. You might consider the last couple of pages to be an ill-judged case of overshare, but explaining my ability to train myself to become depressed is a necessary introduction to a future direction that this book will take—namely, a hypothesis about how psychoses work in Section D: Delusions.

SUMMARY OF COMPULSIVE ACTION STATES

We have now completed the description of basic cases of compound self-destruction in humans that involve mixing two emotions with a single stimulus. You should now recognise this as a 2x2 matrix (four quadrants) that looks like this (Table 5):

TABLE 5: A SUMMARY OF COMPULSIVE ACTION STATES

. . . is the Affectation Stimulus for the behaviour associated with the emotion below	The Biological Stimulus for this emotion . . .	
	Driver 1	Inhibitor 1
Driver 2	A Compulsion: An urge to perform an action, where the performance of that action does not cause the urge to terminate. For example, the constant need to wash your hands.	A Libertine Compulsion: A compulsion to perform an action that is asocial or antisocial. For example, raping or killing.
Inhibitor 2	An Anti-Compulsion: A compulsion to *not* perform an essential action. For example, urination, social interaction or eating.	A Universal Anti-Compulsion: A compulsion to do nothing, possibly extending to a total shutdown of all functionality. For example, catalepsy or waxy flexibility.

I believe that this classificatory system approximately describes the spectrum of psychiatric disorders that psychiatrists used to call 'neurosis'. I have explained that all these symptoms are logically derived, and I believe that this incorporates all forms of compulsion. Maybe I am boasting when I say 'all'. After all, I am not a psychiatrist and I am sure they could tell me of some cases of compulsive self-destruction that do not appear to fit this model. I have not read the entire psychiatric case history. I am a logician, and we do not *do* research; we just place one concept in front of another in a structured sequence of thoughts. However, once you accept that this model demonstrates that a wide range of compulsive action states are rationally derived solely from manipulated behaviour, it seems appropriate to stop calling them 'mental illnesses' or 'mental disorders'. In fact, most of the terms that have been used in the past now seem inappropriate. Some of them are intentionally derogatory anyway. So from now on, I am going to drop all such terminology and, instead, just refer to Compulsions and Anti-Compulsions, whether they are Libertine, Universal or not. We now have a causal mechanism, so we should stop thinking of these problems just in terms of symptoms or effects.

Anyone who has any experience with mathematics will recognise that we could carry on from here. We could extrapolate this idea to an infinite degree, starting with an exploration of three emotions getting tangled together, but I am not going to do this now. There is a danger of getting carried away with a mathematical extrapolation when a human may well only be able to consider a small number of emotional variables at once. There may well be some people whose madness is so severe that they are indeed confusing three or more variables simultaneously. But we need to learn to walk before we can run, and we still have not completed the description of all the possible ways that just two emotions can become confused.

C:
IMPULSIONS

Science may be described as the art of
systematic over-simplification—the art of
discerning what we may with advantage omit.
— Karl Popper, The Open Universe

A THOUGHT AS A STIMULUS FOR ACTION

In Section B: Compulsions, we considered hypothetical people who get muddled up between two emotions because the behaviour associated with one emotion was replaced with that of another. Our subjects took the Biological Stimulus of one emotion to be the Affectation Stimulus for another. This resulted in them misunderstanding two emotions simultaneously. Here in Section C: Impulsions, we are going to consider hypothetical people who are also confused about which emotion is which, not because the behaviour is inverted or affected, but because the behaviour for both has been suppressed. Our subjects are therefore missing the marker for identification of two emotions. I hope to demonstrate that this can give rise to patterns of deviant proactive response to situations that should be prompted by one of the emotions. This results in a different outcome to what we explored in Section B, but which can also be tabulated in a structured way.

To recap: a biological emotion is a function that converts a set of circumstances into an action state. This function has been honed to perfection by 3 billion years of evolution by natural selection to optimise your survival in all circumstances. And we are concerned with how humans can confuse this by trying to out-think their own biology. Almost all people manipulate the behaviour associated with a particular emotion for some particular stimulus. This is always ultimately self-destructive to some degree, but we all tend to survive it if it is marginal or non-systemic, or because we have other mechanisms for survival that have arrived in the last nanosecond of evolutionary time, like houses that prevent predators eating us and fire that prevents us dying of cold. The thesis of this book is that madness is self-destruction squared because we are combining two such effects together.

Compulsion arises because a Biological Stimulus, which is misidentified, leads to an action state that does not counteract that stimulus, so it never switches off. What we need to consider is aberrant action states that are repeating, but not compulsive. These cannot be caused by a Biological Stimulus for an emotion or they would result in another compulsive action state. That leaves us with a problem: what is there in your world that is not a Biological Stimulus for some action or other?

Let us consider a negligible stimulus: you are sitting in your garden and a leaf falls off a tree. When this happens, there is a flicker of movement in your peripheral vision, so your eyes dart towards the stimulus before you revert to whatever you were doing before. The urge to do this arises because your forest dwelling ancestors in the distant evolutionary past had to check that every falling leaf was not a swooping vampire bat or a poisonous spider descending on its web. We could say that the dart of your eyes is a vanishingly small response to a vanishingly small stimulus. We should properly call this an emotional response—albeit a vanishingly small one—since it is a function that turns a set of circumstances: a flicker in your peripheral vision, into an action state: a dart of your eyes. Normally, we would not think of that as an emotional response because it is so negligible, and so we do not have a common name for it. Some people might say that it was not an emotional response, but a reflex. But I am concerned with biological mechanisms that turn sets of circumstances into action states. We do not think of the reflex to withdraw a hand from a snapping dog as an emotional response, but maybe that's just because the response is necessarily too fast for us to try to out-think it. Anger is usually considered an emotion, and one that often has a rapid response, but sometimes we out-think it and sometimes not. We do not think of the reflexive dart of the eyes as an emotional response because it is too negligible for us to bother out-thinking it. However, we are capable of out-thinking any response. I once knew a girl who trained herself to fall downstairs while suppressing the urge to reach out with her hand to break her fall. Why? You may well ask. And to that, I have no answer. Maybe the ancient Roman, Gaius Mucius Scaevola, would be a good person to ask, since he intentionally burnt off his right hand to demonstrate how little he cared for his body.

Let us return to the dart of the eyes when a leaf falls from a tree. Suppose that you suppress the emotional response to this infinitesimal stimulus—maybe because you think you are too cool. This is actually infinitesimally self-destructive because in your infinite future (should you otherwise live that long) you will be killed by the bite of a poisonous spider or a rabid vampire bat that you did not see coming. Practically everything in your world is a stimulus to which biology programmes you to have a response. And you can out-think practically every such response—assuming that you have the time, can be bothered and can see some tactical advantage in doing so. This means that in our search for the stimulus for any other type of repetitive inappropriate action, we need to discard Biological Stimuli for other emotions because that simply results in us repeating the analysis of Section B. And since almost everything in your physical environment is a Biological Stimulus of some sort, we need to ignore all external stimuli. We therefore need to consider internal stimuli for the hypothetical situation that we are trying to create—namely thoughts. But what sort of thought is relevant?

IDENTIFYING AN EMOTION

Wittgenstein starts his *Philosophical Investigations* with a quote from Augustine:

> When they (my elders) named some object, and accordingly moved towards something, I saw this and I grasped that the thing was called by the sound they uttered when they meant to point it out. Their intention was shown by the bodily movements, as it were the natural language of all peoples: the expression of the face, the play of the eyes, the movement of other parts of the body, and the tone of voice which expresses our state of mind in seeking, having, rejecting, or avoiding something. Thus, as I heard words repeatedly used in their proper places in various sentences, I gradually learnt to understand what objects they signified: and after I had trained my mouth to form these signs, I used them to express my own desires.[102]

Wittgenstein says that this accurately reflects how we grasp simple noun words like 'table', 'chair', 'bread', but the story is a little more complex for verbs, colours, concept words such as numbers, and expressions like 'this thing' and 'approximately there'. He then creates a theory of language based around the analogy of games, where the rules must be followed, but they shift depending upon the context.

What I intend to do is to follow his method but focus solely upon how we understand words for emotions and form concepts of them. We need to understand how this process is supposed to work because then, when we imagine hypothetically corrupting elements of the process, we can make deductions about how this understanding would itself be corrupted. My aim is to explain how a human can misidentify his or her own emotion and then explore what the consequences of this would be. It is my contention that by doing this, we can create a theoretical map describing the spectrum of psychiatric conditions generally known as 'acute personality disorders'. Psychiatrists do not understand the causal structure of acute personality disorders. There are several theories,[103] but these show little convergence on consensus—partly, I suspect, because they are framed with many nebulous concepts like 'secondary emotions', 'learned anxiety', 'maternal implanting', etc., that themselves do not have agreed causal structures. This makes such theories impossible to test empirically; so none of them can be refuted. Consider how you would set up an experiment that demonstrated that a human (with the added complexity of a mental disorder) experienced secondary emotions or had learned anxiety. It is this difficulty that makes such theories speculative. It is arguable that they are not even scientific hypotheses.

My approach differs from most other theorists in that I do not examine mentally ill people from a top-down process by trying to understand what is going on with them. Instead, I construct pure theory from a bottom-up process by breaking down the concept of an emotion into its component parts, explaining how we understand that concept, and then taking away the inputs necessary to that understanding to derive a description of a mistaken understanding of an emotion. We can then ask how a person with such an incorrect understanding should be expected to act—assuming they are rational. Once we have thus broken down all the possibilities, we can overlay that map against the empirical observations of psychiatrists who have described the various forms of acute personality disorder. I hope to demonstrate that this process produces an approximate fit. If this fit is agreed, then we have a concrete hypothesis of how acute personality disorder works.

If we are trying to explain how we understand emotions, a good place to start is to imagine that we are trying to teach a small child the words for them. When a child does something naughty, the father reacts and the mother says 'your father is angry'. As she says this, she refers by pointing or gesturing at the father. But she is clearly communicating to the child some attribute of the father. One of the great mysteries of language is that children, from a very young age, have no difficulty distinguishing between an object and an attribute of that object. The attribute in question is anger and the child is being referred by the mother to something about the father that is different from normal. And that thing is a behavioural state.

If there is no behavioural state, there can be no word for anger because there would be nothing that we could see. So, in the sense that Augustine describes pointing at something and uttering a sound, what would we point at? That is the biological purpose of the behavioural state. It is a signalling mechanism that is fundamental to communication between social animals and it has its origin in evolution by natural selection. Anger is observable in social animals that cannot speak and have no words for it. If we study it in chimpanzees, we can see that it has two generic triggers: firstly, another chimpanzee fails to perform a social obligation (e.g. grooming fleas); or, secondly, it performs an antisocial action (e.g. stealing food). It should be noted that each of these generic triggers is itself a pretty wide class of actions. Anger has consequences that are themselves emotional: in the first instance, it triggers guilt in the chimpanzee that did not perform its duty and this drives the performance of onerous social obligations; and, in the second instance, it triggers shame that inhibits the performance of antisocial actions.

When we first teach a child the word 'anger' we usually do it by pointing to the behaviour of another person, so that behaviour is a prerequisite of understanding. As Wittgenstein puts it:

'What would it be like if human beings showed no outward signs of pain (did not groan, grimace, etc.)? Then it would be impossible to teach a child the use of the word 'tooth-ache'.' – Well, let's assume the child is a genius and itself invents a name for the sensation! – But then, of course, he couldn't make himself understood when he used the word. – So does he understand the name, without being able to explain its meaning to anyone? – But what does it mean to say that he has 'named his pain'? – How has he done this naming of pain?! And whatever he did, what was its purpose? – When one says: 'He gave a name to his sensation' one forgets that a great deal of stage-setting in the language is presupposed if the mere act of naming is to make sense. And when we speak of someone's having given a name to pain, what is presupposed is the existence of the grammar of the word 'pain'; it shows the post where the new word is stationed.[104]

Wittgenstein extends this argument to a whole host of other sensations and the words associated with them, such as the sensation of seeing a colour or thinking about a number. But I want to stick with sensations connected to emotions. And then I want to take the argument on a detour that Wittgenstein did not take. I want to explore the impact of selective suppression of the behaviour. Wittgenstein almost went down this road when he says of pain:

That expression of doubt has no place in the language-game; but if we cut out human behaviour, which is the expression of sensation, it looks as if I might legitimately begin to doubt afresh. My temptation to say that one might take a sensation for something other than what it is arises from this: if I assume the abrogation of the normal language-game with the expression of a sensation, I need a criterion of identity for the sensation; and then the possibility of error also exists.[105]

Science, these days, is only interested in what can be empirically demonstrated. Since feelings cannot be measured, nothing scientific can be said about them other than the scientist telling us that he experiences them. Psychologists therefore do not really talk about feelings much and it is now generally accepted that feelings have no place in psychological theories. But that is not to say that they are meaning-less. As Wittgenstein puts it:

> 'But doesn't what you say come to this: that there is no pain, for example, without pain-behaviour?' – It comes to this: only of a living human being and what resembles (behaves like) a living human being can one say: it has sensations; it sees; is blind; hears; is deaf; is conscious or unconscious.[106]

Consider a surgical operation where the anaesthetist makes a mistake: the anaesthetic stopped the patient being able to move or cry out, but did not make them unconscious. The surgeon cuts them open without realising that they can feel extraordinary pain because they have no way of indicating this pain. Clearly, in this case, the sensation matters; not the behaviour or the word for it! We might ask (as some indeed do) whether a plant can feel pain. But this makes no sense in evolutionary terms: a pain that has no behaviour or no result-ing action has no function in the process of survival or reproduction. How, then, would the complex neurological (or other) processes that presumably are required for registering pain come into being? We can imagine that a frog feels pain even though it does not have human-like behavioural representation because it takes avoiding actions (unlike a plant). This gives us a clue that it feels pain but no certainty.

Behaviour is not a prerequisite of the sensation of pain, but it is a prerequisite of our ability to recognise it in another person (or animal with human-like behaviour) and to give it a name. Wittgen-stein uses pain as his example because it serves the purpose of his analysis well. Pain is easy to understand because it reliably results from certain types of injury; the behaviour is pretty consistent; and generally nobody performs tactical deception with this behaviour. And if (hypothetically) you really do not understand what pain is, I can demonstrate it to you easily by pricking you with a pin—this of course presumes that you are not immune to pain due to some strange neurological condition or suchlike. Pain is a good introduction to this way of thinking, but I want to extrapolate this to anger. With anger, we have some added complications. Firstly, you or I might come from a family or culture where the suppression of the behaviour of anger is commonplace; and, secondly, if (hypothetically) you do not understand what anger is, I do not have a comparable way of demonstrating it to you like pricking you with a pin. If I try to demonstrate it to you by doing something purely to make you angry, then the knowledge that I am doing it purely for those purposes would naturally mean that you would not be angry anyway.

Let us return to the child whose parents are teaching it the word for anger. The first step is pointing out anger in another person—in the example I used, the father. This necessarily involves referring to the behaviour—the only part of anger in another person that can be seen by anybody else. The second step requires the child to lose its temper itself. The parent can then say 'why are you angry?' The child now has the means to connect their response to that of another person. A word only has meaning when two people understand it the same way and use it to communicate. For two people to understand the word 'anger', it is necessary that they both, at some point, display the behaviour.

On another occasion, a parent might ask the child 'are you *feeling* angry?' Here we are introducing to the child a new concept. But what are we to make of it? The parent cannot see the child's feelings, they just suppose that they are there. But what is there? What is its nature? This is an unanswerable question, but it does not matter that it is unanswerable. When a primatologist studies chimpanzees and notices that they jump up and down and scream when another acts in a way that disadvantages them, the primatologist concludes that the chimpanzee is angry based upon its human-like behaviour and the circumstances that provoked the behaviour. There is nothing to be gained from wondering what the chimpanzee *feels*. We can draw a diagram (Figure 9) of an emotion like this:

FIGURE 9: A SIMPLE REPRESENTATION OF THE WORKING OF AN EMOTION

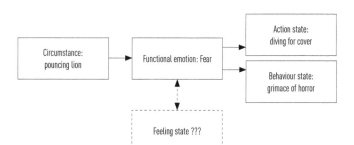

... and the purpose of all the causal elements are pretty straightforward (both to scientists and non-scientists) except for the part denoted by dotted lines. What is the feeling? Does it even exist? Does the emotion cause the feeling or vice versa? Without the feeling, is there no emotion? The point is that the function of the emotion is complete even when we ignore the dotted line box, so why do we need to worry about it? Of course, we could argue that without the feeling, we would not know that we had to dive for cover, but that still does not tell us what it is. A ringing bell or a red flashing light in our heads could serve the same purpose. Alternatively (and more realistically) a bunch of neurones interact to create the response, and somehow we have a conscious awareness of this. But this awareness is just a specific instance of the wider problem of consciousness. Nobody knows what it is—and that includes both scientists and philosophers. Take one of the fastest responses: the withdrawal of your hand from a burning surface. You cannot say that the pain makes you do this. It happens far too fast for you to even think about it. Your pain receptor nerve fires into your brain and your brain fires the nerve to the muscles in your arm that makes your hand withdraw, and all of that happens before you even have the conscious experience of the pain. We often call this a reflex, but the only difference between this and any other action is that it happens too fast for us to second-guess it?

What I have been seeking to demonstrate is that we can still talk meaningfully about emotions as biological functions when we completely ignore the dotted line box. The complete understanding of an emotion requires us to: 1) know what circumstances cause it; 2) know what action results; and 3) know what its name is. The latter is only necessary if we want to talk about it (which most of us do). If we know all these elements, we do not need to know what it feels like—although most of us consider that to be its essence. As Wittgenstein puts it:

> We ask 'What does "I am frightened" really mean, what am I referring to when I say it?' And of course we find no answer, or one that is inadequate.[107]

He then goes on to say:

> What is fear? What does 'being afraid' mean? If I wanted to define it in a *single* showing, I would *play-act* fear.[108]

The only way to explain it is to mimic the behaviour, and the statement 'I know I have feelings because I can feel them' is incoherent and explains nothing. (Comparison: 'I know I have zarkings because I can zark them.' Refute *that*!)

Let us now intentionally corrupt this process. I am using anger as my example because it is an emotion for which the behaviour is commonly suppressed. Assume that we consider another small child that grows up in a family that systematically suppresses the behaviour associated with anger. Not only are such families common, I can think of cultures where everybody does this—India and Bali spring to mind. The first step of our learning process: 'your father is angry' is going to be missing in such a family—or at least the mother will say that to the child without having any behaviour to point at. The child is unlikely to be first introduced to the concept by the behaviour of another. We then have to consider what the parent says when the child itself loses its temper. At the first instance, the child has no way of knowing that displaying such behaviour is frowned upon, since it has never encountered it; so it will not suppress the behaviour. Suppressing behaviour, when it is a cultural norm (even if only within the family), needs to be learned. When the child loses its temper in the first instance, we could imagine that the parent would ask 'why are you angry?' just like in our original example. But what if, because anger is considered to be an undesirable emotional state, the parent says 'such behaviour is *shameful!*'? Here we are laying the foundations, not only for removing the basis for being able to recognise an emotion within oneself, but also for implanting the idea that an emotion of one type is actually another. We are exploring a simple mechanism whereby an ordinary human that does not have anything functionally wrong with their neurological brain can misidentify their own emotion.

Let us consider the proposition: 'I know that I am angry because I can feel it' and apply it in these circumstances. How does a person raised in such circumstances know that what they feel is anger? The feeling—assuming that we have an inkling of its metaphysics—does not come with a label attached to it. The only means of identifying it is behaviour, both in ourselves and in others. The behaviour is the link that enables us to make the connection between the word associated with an emotion and its supposed feeling. We have created a hypothetical circumstance where this link is broken. How can anybody know what anger is supposed to feel like if they cannot feel anybody else's? Even if anger does have a feeling, and we give it a name, we can only attach the correct name if everybody is displaying the correct behaviour.

If you doubt this analysis, consider another problem: let us agree that there are two ways of identifying an emotion—what it looks like (behaviour) and what it *feels* like (sensation). Now, we have to assume that the feeling is something that we can remember consistently—like I can remember what the colour red looks like. I have explained elsewhere[109] that although we can remember simple colours quite well, we tend to overestimate our ability to remember subtle differences in shades—generally we misremember them. We can demonstrate that we misremember because we can subsequently reference a colour card to remind ourselves. It is usually a mistake to buy a blue tie thinking it will go nicely with a blue shirt that is at home in your wardrobe because when you put them together the blues will likely clash—you fail to remember the shade accurately. If we misremember a feeling, there is no equivalent to the colour card, so how can we ever know whether we misremembered? Nobody else can correct us because nobody else can know what we are feeling. If we cannot know that we misremembered, then clearly we have no way of knowing that we remembered correctly either. If I try to remember a historical experience of one of my own emotions, I am actually not sure I can recall any feeling—I can recall the behaviour associated with the emotion and that creates a false belief in me that I am recalling the feeling. Try to remember what pain feels like without recalling an image of a grimace! I am sure you will find it is harder than you think.

Here is another analogy. Assume you ask me for directions to the post office and I just invent the directions for my own amusement. It is rational for you to follow my directions until it becomes clear that they are a nonsense fabrication. Now assume that I mislead you by pretending with my behaviour. What is the equivalent moment of discovery? Describe what you might experience at such a moment? What does that moment *feel* like?

Another huge complication is that a child gobbles up language effortlessly; but an adult learning a foreign language has to rote-learn every word and then be force-fed the grammar. Assume that a child mislearned an emotion word because they grew up in a family that manipulated the behaviour. How would we address this when that mislearned word started to affect them in adult life? This would be like learning a foreign language without a dictionary.

What I intend to do in this part of the book is explore the consequences of the misidentification of emotions due to suppressed behaviour. I take shame to be an inhibitor that prevents antisocial actions and guilt to be a driver of onerous social obligations, but sometimes in normal parlance we use these words interchangeably. We could easily get lost in a worthless conversation about what these two words mean rather than discussing the nature of what the words refer to. The fundamental problem here is that I am a person who is confused about *my* emotions, explaining to you—a person who is presumably confused about *your* emotions—why it is that all humans are confused about *their* emotions. This is a less-than-ideal place to begin an intellectual journey! It is easy for us to lose our way upon taking the first step; so, to avoid this, I am going to continue with the abstract language from Section B: Compulsions. I am going to explore hypothetical emotions that I call 'Driver' and 'Inhibitor'. And, as in the prior discussion of compulsive actions, there are four possible ways that we can get the identities of driving and inhibiting emotions confused:

1. Driver 1 is mistaken for Driver 2.
2. Inhibitor is mistaken for Driver.
3. Driver is mistaken for Inhibitor.
4. Inhibitor 1 is mistaken for Inhibitor 2.

DEVIANT PROACTION

L et us consider a generic driving emotion that I am going to call 'Driver 1'. We can describe it in the following diagram (Figure 10):

FIGURE 10: GENERIC DIAGRAM OF A SUPPRESSED DRIVING EMOTION

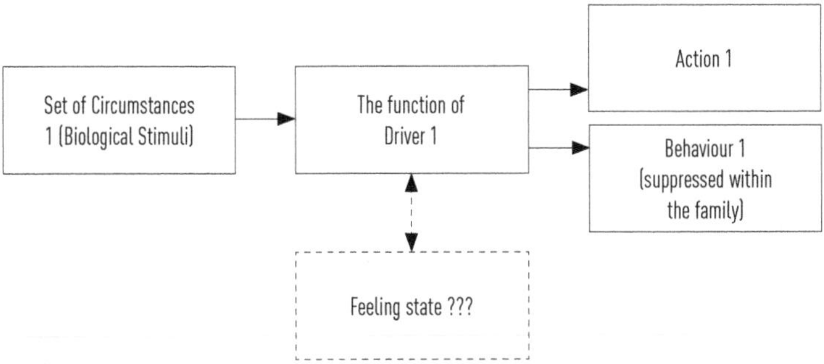

... except we are going to imagine that we are considering a girl who was raised in a family where the behaviour associated with Driver 1 was suppressed systematically. This may have arisen because her family thought such behaviour was shameful or a sign of weakness, but why it happens does not really matter much for the purposes of this thought experiment.

When she first encountered the emotion in herself, naturally the behaviour would follow—a child will not suppress behaviour unless it has a reason to do so. But the family will express shock at the behavioural display (because it is shameful or a sign of weakness) and so she will learn to suppress it too.

Her family is not an island. It lives in a world where there are other people who do not think that there is anything wrong with displaying this behaviour. Her parents might tell her that a person in the street who displays Behaviour 1 is experiencing the emotion that we are calling Driver 1. ('Tsk, tsk!') Her parents might explain that this occurred because of a specific instance of a Biological Stimuli within set of Circumstances 1 and she can see this person in the street performing Action 1. She will therefore have a word for it 'Driver 1' and she can identify the emotion in other people via the behaviour. Her concept of it could even be pretty complete from the perspective of her observing it in other people (outside her family). Note that the set of circumstances that serve as Biological Stimuli for Driver 1 might be quite wide, and if she does not see this behaviour within her own family, she may only have an awareness of a limited subset of this totality. Also note that her family may only suppress the behaviour for just a subset of the total set of such Biological Stimuli, so again she would have an understanding of Driver 1, but maybe not the complete set of circumstances that normally trigger it. Mostly, I am going to describe binary misconceptions of emotions—purely for simplicity, but we should remember that misconceptions can vary by minute degrees. This situation, results in her growing up with an impaired ability to identify this emotion *in herself* because it can only be identified via the behaviour—and this is missing (wholly or in part) in herself because she has been trained to suppress it.

Now let us assume that exactly the same thing happens to this girl with respect to another emotion that I will call 'Driver 2'. So the girl has an ability to understand this emotion in other people (outside the family)—she has a limited understanding of the set of Circumstances 2, but recognises Action 2 and Behaviour 2. Again, she has a greatly impaired ability to identify it in herself.

Let us say that the emotion Driver 1 arises in her in adolescence. Let us also assume that it is triggered by a circumstance that she has not encountered before and where she has never seen this circumstance cause Driver 1 in people in the street. If no behaviour arises because she has been trained to suppress it, then she will not know that it is Driver 1. But it is an intense experience, nonetheless—perhaps one that is slightly alarming. Let us say, that because of something suggested to her in her childhood, she imagines that she is experiencing 'Driver 2'—also an emotion where she has been trained to suppress the behaviour.

What are the consequences of this new situation?

It would be easy to imagine that this particular instance from the set of Circumstances 1 would cause Action 2. However, if this is the first time that she has experienced this, it would give rise to just one instance of doing something strange. All of us have had at least one instance in our lives of a strange response to an unfamiliar situation, but that does not result in our being diagnosed with an acute personality disorder. A therapist might pick up on it and ask her 'why did you do Action 2 instead of Action 1?' Training her in the realignment of her responses would be relatively simple. But this is a human with an enhanced ability to understand her own emotions (and therefore misunderstand them), and in particular an ability to understand future emotions. She is not a survival machine, but a machine that goal-seeks emotional outcomes. The emotion does not drive the action; instead, she calculates the action to engineer her emotional outcome. For example, humans do not wait until they are hungry before they seek food like a chimpanzee does; they can predict future hunger, so they seek food in advance to strategise its avoidance.

This woman (now that she is an adult) is going to perform Action 2, whenever she is concerned that this instance of Circumstance 1 might arise in the imminent future. This concern is merely a thought—an expectation. She performs this proactively to try to strategise her emotional outcome, but she is performing the calculation incorrectly because she has misidentified the emotion whose outcome she is trying to strategise and therefore she is confused about the emotional goal. The result is an action inappropriate to her situation that does not require any Biological Stimulus to trigger it.

For a therapist, it is difficult to work out this trigger because it is a thought that cannot be seen. And the patient cannot explain the thought because it is itself a misunderstanding.

Before we move on, it is perhaps helpful to briefly compare the situation just described above to the situation described earlier in Section B: Compulsions under A Compulsion to Perform an Action. There we also encountered a person who confuses one emotion with another. Why is this situation different? In the earlier case, the emotions (emotions 4 and 7) were confused because the Biological Stimulus for one emotion (emotion 4) became the Affectation Stimulus for another (emotion 7). This resulted in an action state that did not negate the Biological Stimulus so it never switched off. If the behaviour is the sign for the emotion, it is a *certainty* that the wrong behaviour is going to result in deducing the identity of your emotion incorrectly. In this case, the woman is confused because *no* behaviour is on display and she has no means of identifying either in herself. It is little more than a random coin-toss that she is going to identify one or both of them incorrectly. This is a situation that could be open to all sorts of suggestibility that arose as she grew up. One such example is that of a parent in a family that suppresses anger saying 'such behaviour is shameful' when the child displays anger behaviour. For now, we are going to ignore this possibility in this instance for the purposes of stripping the idea down to its simplest elements. This new situation is *not* a compulsion, but a proactive calculation of an action (that is normally the outcome of the emotion Driver 2) to prevent a predicted future emotional state that most people would identify as Driver 1, but that this person is misidentifying. It does not need any Biological Stimulus for this Deviant Proaction to occur—just a thought that is a misconception.

PROACTIVE IMPULSION

Following the pattern of Section B: Compulsions, we can now repeat the analysis assuming that another hypothetical person mistakes an emotion 'Driver 1' for one that I will call 'Inhibitor 3'. The Driver is the same as either Driver 1 or 2 in the previous chapter, but Inhibitor 3 can be described in the following diagram (Figure 11):

FIGURE 11: GENERIC DIAGRAM OF A SUPPRESSED INHIBITING EMOTION

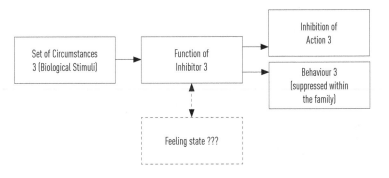

This is an emotion that inhibits a particular set of actions that I call collectively 'Action 3' upon a particular set of circumstances. For example, the emotional inhibitor of tiredness inhibits physical activity upon the body accumulating lactic acid or depleted energy levels; and the emotional inhibitor of shame inhibits the performance of antisocial actions in circumstances where you can take advantage of someone else's weakness.

As before, we are going to imagine that we are considering a boy who was raised in a family where the behaviour associated with each emotion (Behaviour 1 and Behaviour 3) were suppressed throughout his formative years. At some point in his adolescence, this boy has an experience where he encounters a stimulus that resides in the set of Circumstances 3 that he has never encountered before. His reaction to this is strong, but he cannot understand it, so he starts to wonder whether what he is experiencing is an instance of Driver 1. The biological purpose of Inhibitor 3 is to stop him performing whatever action he was thinking of performing the moment it arose.

As an adult, the boy—now a man—will calculate his actions to achieve emotional goals. He buys food to circumvent future hunger, he plans vacations to strategise future contentment and he gains professional qualifications to avoid anxiety about his future wellbeing. To achieve these simple human tasks without going off the rails, he needs to be able to correctly identify his emotions and what causes them. But there is one instance where he is not doing this correctly. Inhibitor 3 is a biological function that inhibits action, including antisocial actions. He has a poor ability to identify this emotion in himself and he has an incomplete understanding of all the circumstances that cause it. In particular, there is one circumstance that most of us recognise falls into the set of Circumstances 3 that cause Inhibitor 3. Most of us, trying to engineer our emotional outcomes will inhibit whatever action we are considering performing, but this man will calculate that he should perform Action 1 proactively to engineer an emotional outcome, since he thinks that he is trying to circumvent a future occurrence of the emotion of Driver 1.

He proactively calculates Action 1 where he should be calculating that the correct response is to inhibit action. We have now described a situation where a mere thought—an expectation of a future set of circumstances—gives rise to a proactive calculation that he should act in circumstances that require constraint—a Proactive Impulsion. The result is a pattern of obnoxious, impulsive, imprudent or antisocial actions that do not need a Biological Stimulus to provoke them.

Let us consider possibly the most destructive way that a misidentification of this nature can occur: a man confuses shame with humiliation. This is not too hard to imagine because sometimes in casual parlance we use these terms synonymously. But we need to consider their biology to understand just how wrong this is and how destructive the consequences are.

Darwin described the evolution of the humiliation-revenge response in *The Decent of Man*.[110] Female humans invest more in raising their children (including pregnancy and breastfeeding) than male humans, so it is more important to a female human that the child is strong. Bluntly put, a man that invests nothing in the raising of his child has no reason to care if that child thrives. That means that females tend to be extremely careful to select male breeding partners with strong gene sets, but males are comparatively unselective—particularly when they have no intention of assisting in the nurturing of offspring. Biologists call species with this asymmetric sexual selection a 'polygynous' species. Women are selective, and that means that men of high social status are more likely to have offspring than men of low social status. But men are less selective, so women have the same prospects of having offspring whether they are of high or low social status. This is pure evolutionary theory that is entirely supported by empirical observations. The effect is enhanced when we look at primitive tribal societies, where village chiefs often practice polygamy and dominate breeding rights. In nature, we can find species, such as red deer and elephant seals that are highly polygynous. Here almost all offspring in any year are fathered by a tiny minority of the pool of males of breeding age. These males are large, strong and pugnacious. For a male who fails to breed, in evolutionary terms it is equivalent to dying, which explains why males fight over breeding rights—occasionally to death. If we apply these principles to humans it explains why human males are approximately 50 times as likely to kill another male as a human female is to kill another female; why male homicide is statistically biased towards early adulthood—the age when men are seeking breeding partners; and why homicide is statistically biased towards men of low social status. These statistics are pretty consistent for every society from urban America to tribal societies in the forests of Papua New Guinea.[111] Humiliation is a biological emotion where the Biological Stimulus is a threat to breeding rights (or in biologist-speak 'biological fitness') and the action that results is an attack on the source of the threat. Such an attack is called a 'revenge response', and humiliation is therefore a driving emotion.

Shame is an inhibiting emotion that prevents humans performing antisocial actions. But do shame and humiliation *feel* the same or different? It is not insignificant that the words for these emotions are occasionally used synonymously, like 'shame' and 'guilt' are often used synonymously. A person who is confusing shame with humiliation will turn any situation that should provoke inhibition into an attack. Although no psychiatric professional body officially endorses the term as a name for a diagnosis, this disorder is commonly known as 'psychopathy', particularly in forensic psychology—an acute personality disorder that makes such people impossible to manage outside of a prison. This is a typical example of Proactive Impulsion. Note that it is commonly thought that psychopaths do not have feelings towards others. I believe that this is a mistake. They have feelings, but they misidentify what they are.

It is worth pointing out here, that psychopathy is a completely different mechanism to a Libertine Compulsion, which could lead to serial killers and child molesters being compulsive without being psychopathic. True serial killers are quite rare, but most prisons in the Western world are overflowing with people (particularly men) who have Proactive Impulsion—particularly antisocial personality disorder. I will discuss this more later, but I believe that antisocial personality disorder is a Proactive Impulsion that results from a person misidentifying their emotion of shame as anger.

DEVIANT ANTI-IMPULSION

Again, repeating the pattern of Section B: Compulsions, if we can mistake an inhibiting emotion for a driving emotion, we can clearly do it the other way round. The outcome should by now be pretty obvious. Such a person is going to convert anticipated situations that would normally prompt proactive action and into aversion to action. Whatever results, if it occurs in circumstances when others would be proactive, it will appear to be unreasonably inhibited. I call this 'Deviant Anti-Impulsion'.

Let us consider an example. Although psychiatrists are unclear about the causality of acute personality disorder, one common experience of sufferers of many such conditions is childhood sexual abuse or other traumatic experience. In particular, studies have shown that people who were verbally abused in childhood were three times more likely to manifest borderline, narcissistic, obsessive-compulsive or paranoid personality disorders.[112] However, socio-economic factors also have a considerable bearing on some outcomes (particularly paranoid, schizoid, schizotypal and passive-aggressive personality disorders).[113] We can now explain a hypothesis as to how traumatic experience can give rise to a Deviant Anti-Impulsion. The diagram in Figure 12 (which I have used before) describes an emotion that few of us would have difficulty understanding:

FIGURE 12: DIAGRAM OF A DRIVING EMOTION

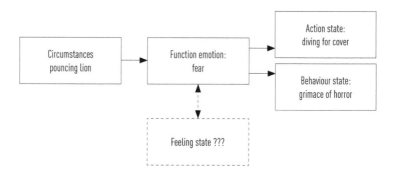

Now consider the following diagram (Figure 13) of a complex emotional situation by way of comparison. All of the boxes belong in dotted lines because none of the causal linkages are clear, either to the subject or to their therapist:

FIGURE 13: AN APPARENT INHIBITING EMOTION ARISING FROM A MEMORY

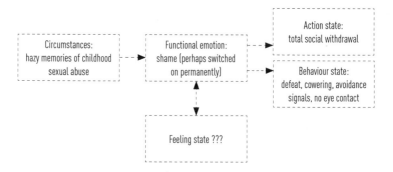

We also need to consider that the memories of abuse might be false or imagined which is why this situation presents an enigma to anybody who attempts to help such a person, either in a private or professional capacity. You may have avoided childhood abuse on this scale, but most of us had some emotional experience that was inexplicable.

A complete understanding of an emotion requires us to understand *all* of the circumstances that trigger it. But we all have finite experience. We can extrapolate from this experience to imagine other triggers that we have not encountered ourselves, but this is an imperfect exercise. I may imagine that I know what the experience of famine is like because I once skipped two meals in a row. But how realistic is that? What my extrapolation is missing is the understanding of which parts of the experience you can adapt to and which you cannot. When you have a traumatic experience, it is probable that you have a reaction that you have never observed in another person. Clearly, the biological reaction should be to cry out and run away. But what if you could not do this—either because you are a soldier in a foxhole or because your sexual molester is sitting on your chest. You have an intense emotional experience with a suppression of the natural response to that experience. Therefore, you are likely to have an inability to identify that emotion correctly. The knowledge that the experience belittles you as a person, means that you do not want to talk about it. And this makes it easy to misidentify the emotion as shame. A driver (fear) is misidentified as an inhibitor (shame). And for the rest of such a person's life, the natural concern that the experience could reoccur, could lead to a Deviant Anti-Impulsion. We now have a worked example of how a traumatic life experience can cause an acute personality disorder without it requiring any Biological Stimulus or any dysfunction with the biological brain.

DEVIANT RESTRAINT VS NON-DEVIANT RESTRAINT?

In Section B: Compulsions, I explained that we can invert the behaviour associated with two inhibiting emotions and cause an outcome that I called the Universal Anti-Compulsion. Is there an equivalent mechanism here? Let us suppose that a person confuses one inhibiting emotion (Inhibitor 1) with another (Inhibitor 2) because the behaviour associated with both has been suppressed, then in a situation where they are supposed to *not* do something, they will not do that thing for the wrong reason.

Uh! . . . So What?

Let us suppose that the emotion of shame is supposed to stop you stealing an old lady's handbag. But you are misidentifying the emotion of shame as another inhibitor: tiredness. Then you do not steal the handbag, not due to moral restraint, but because you cannot be bothered. And what exactly is the observable dysfunction here when considered from the perspective of action?

It is nicely elegant, mathematically, if we mix two variables together in all possible combinations and end up with four theoretical results. But, sadly, in this case the fourth theoretical result is a dud and not something of interest to psychiatrists. Maybe that is a good thing because we have enough mental disorders to cope with and do not need any more. However, it is not a problem that we have only three theoretical structures: Deviant Proaction, Proactive Impulsion and Deviant Anti-Impulsion, resulting from this analysis because . . .

MAPPING ACUTE PERSONALITY DISORDER

. . . the APA classifies acute personality disorders into three main groups or 'clusters'. I have mentioned before that it is astonishing how much psychiatry got right without any theory of causality. That is because being pre-scientific does not mean being unscientific. Psychiatry has spent centuries classifying madness without any agreed causal theory and mostly they got the right answers.

Confusing two emotions, because the behaviour has been switched, results in certain misidentification that causes four distinct types of compulsive action state. But confusing them because the behaviour has been suppressed for both emotions, results in patterns of deviant proactive responses to anticipated circumstances. In the latter case, the response is to an expectation or a thought, and not to an external stimulus. As with compulsive actions, for impulsive actions we have a 2x2 matrix (Table 6) that looks like this:

TABLE 6: SUMMARY OF IMPULSIONS

. . . is misidentified as this . .	This emotion . . .	
	Driver 1	Inhibitor 1
Driver 2	Deviant Proaction: a person computes a proactive response that is not appropriate to the circumstances they face.	Proactive Impulsion: a person converts situations requiring restraint into proactions that others perceive as antisocial or impulsive.
Inhibitor 2	Deviant Anti-Impulsion: a person converts a situation requiring proaction into an inhibition of action.	A person does not do something that they should not do, but for the wrong reason. This does not cause any inappropriate action.

Of the three mechanisms I described there is an approximate mapping onto the three clusters of acute personality disorders. But the APA draws their distinctions based on what the symptoms look like, whereas I make them based upon what the structures are, so we have some differences of opinion. I am not a psychiatrist (in case you had forgotten), so I do not have their skills in diagnosis. However, what I am attempting here is effectively to put a diagnosis on a logic model. It is not clear whether a psychiatrist or a logician is better qualified for this task, so I will approach this as a cautious introductory sketch without attempting too much detail. Of the ten acute personality disorders recognised by the APA (paranoid, schizoid, schizotypal, antisocial, borderline, histrionic, narcissistic, avoidant, dependent and obsessive-compulsive), nine of them appear to me to fit this model fairly well, but for schizotypal personality disorder I have doubts. I also subdivide the APA classification of antisocial personality disorder by separating it from psychopathic personality disorder since I believe that these two are distinct. The cumulative effect is that I end up with the same number of acute personality disorders that fit into the model as the APA's classification, but I have added one (psychopathic) and taken away one (schizotypal). In each case I suggest which emotions (whether drivers or inhibitors) are being misidentified, so I am able to describe these mechanisms quite precisely. However, for some of the acute personality disorders that fit the Deviant Proaction model, I am uncertain of one of the driving emotions being misidentified.

CLUSTER A PERSONALITY DISORDERS

It would appear that Cluster A personality disorders (the odd, bizarre and eccentric cluster) result from a person interpreting a driving emotion as an inhibitor. In general, this cluster fits into the model that I call Deviant Anti-Impulsion. This is particularly the case for paranoid and schizoid personality disorders. However, I doubt that schizotypal personality disorder fits into any of these models and we should probably reclassify it and seek explanations elsewhere.

PARANOID PERSONALITY DISORDER

The symptoms of this disorder include the following:

- Social inhibition: distrust of others and belief that they are trying to harm you.
- Inhibition in confiding information or trusting others due to unreasonable fear that such information will be used against you.
- Misinterpretation of innocent remarks or non-threatening situations as personal attacks.
- A retaliatory reaction to perceived slights and the result of holding grudges.
- Unsupported belief of infidelity of the spouse or sexual partner.

One possible explanation for this is that the emotion of humiliation—an emotional driver to retaliate against attack against you—is being mistaken for shame—an inhibitor. If we place these variables into the model of Deviant Anti-Impulsion, then any perceived threat to biological fitness (real or not) will result in an inhibition regarding countering that threat without the threat itself being neutralised. Ultimately this leads to total withdrawal because a person sees himself or herself as powerless to counter threats created by other people, including threats that are imagined. I described the evolutionary basis of humiliation, earlier in this section in Proactive Impulsion, and this made it clear that humiliation is an emotion that is partly derived from males protecting their biological fitness by attacking threats to it. If paranoid personality disorder is caused by someone mistaking humiliation with shame, then I would expect this to be a male biased condition. However, we cannot conclusively determine this based upon research done to date.

SCHIZOID PERSONALITY DISORDER

The symptoms of this disorder include inhibition in all social situations and an unwillingness to engage in society on any level, including the following:

- Inhibition in all social situations: preferring to be alone and unable to follow social cues or enjoy hobbies.
- Inhibition in expressing all emotions.
- Inhibition regarding having sex with another person.

We achieve an approximate fit if we assume that this condition arises from the subject identifying their emotion of loneliness—an emotional driver regarding seeking human company—as shame—an inhibitor. If we place these variables into the model of Deviant Anti-Impulsion, then any urge to seek human company will result in an aversion to that company resulting in conflict, but ultimately withdrawal.

The final Cluster A personality disorder is schizotypal personality disorder. The symptoms of this disorder include those of schizoid personality disorder plus a range of bizarre additional ones:

- Unconventional dress, beliefs, speech or behaviour.
- Unsupported perceptual experiences. For example, hearing voices calling the subject's name.
- 'Magical thinking' beliefs that affect actions, resulting in highly unconventional practices—similar to a private religion. Belief that insignificant events have hidden messages that only the subject understands.
- Overly elaborate or metaphorical ways of explaining seemingly simple things.

These additional symptoms, however, do not fit this theory well, and we probably need to search for explanations elsewhere. In *Part II: Irrefutable Thoughts* of *The Logic of Self-Destruction*, I sought to demonstrate that belief in ideology or religion was a logic mechanism. In particular, it resulted from tautologies that arose in a strange way: if a belief causes you to modify your emotional behaviour (and I think it demonstrable that it does) then the belief that the ideology or religion brings about human well-being is irrefutable because the belief causes the behaviour of that well-being. You modify your behaviour to demonstrate your compliance with the ideology or religion and, thereby, create a belief in your own well-being that derives solely from modified behaviour that is itself caused by the belief. I suspect that there are elements of this in schizotypal personality disorder. Either way it has certain symptoms that fit the model of Deviant Anti-Impulsion (such as withdrawal or a shameful response to ordinary situations), but there is far too much going on here for which we need other explanations.

Perhaps the oddness of schizotypal personality disorder is intended to drive away other people and therefore, serves the purpose of repelling human company—the emotional need is avoidance of company and affecting strange behaviour assists this. Laing in his book *The Divided Self* describes the 'Schizoid Type' as a precursor to schizophrenia.[114] If a person feels powerless, then they develop a fantasy reality where they achieve emotional fulfilment that is not achievable in the real world. This fantasy reality is consistent with the bizarre dress and speech, and the magical thinking beliefs. Clearly, this is a different model to the Deviant Anti-Impulsion model.

The World Health Organization's ICD-10 appears to partly agree with Laing, and it specifically disagrees with the DSM that 'schizotypal personality disorder' is a personality disorder at all. Rather, it follows Laing in classifying it alongside schizophrenia. And since it does not appear to fit the model that I have described here I would tend to agree. However, schizotypal personality disorder gets its name from the fact that it shares many symptoms with schizophrenia, a psychosis where delusional beliefs are a core symptom. I will discuss this in Section D: Delusions.

CLUSTER B PERSONALITY DISORDERS

Psychiatrists describe Cluster B personality disorders as the dramatic and erratic cluster, which is based upon a common element of emotional excess. I believe that of the Cluster B personality disorders, antisocial and borderline fit into the spectrum of emotional misidentification that I called Proactive Impulsion. An inhibiting emotion is misidentified as a driving emotion. In a situation that would normally be a Biological Stimulus for an inhibiting emotion, the subject calculates an action that will appear highly inappropriate to the situation. This is usually exhibited as impulsiveness, recklessness or an overly emotional response. But narcissistic and histrionic personality disorders fit into the model that I called Deviant Proaction. A driving emotion is misidentified as another driving emotion leading to proactions that seek to strategise the wrong emotional outcome. I further believe that psychopathic personality disorder is a Proactive Impulsion but should be split from antisocial personality disorder.

ANTISOCIAL PERSONALITY DISORDER

Antisocial personality disorder is closely allied to psychopathic personality disorder—the latter is not an officially recognised diagnosis, but is a commonly used term in forensic psychology. However, people with antisocial personality disorder are most likely to end up in prison because of their persistent tendency towards aggression and hostility. One study found that among prisoners in 12 Western countries, 47 per cent of the men and 21 per cent of the women had antisocial personality disorder.[115] The symptoms include:

- Disregard for others' needs or feelings. This could be interpreted as disregard for the inhibiting effect of other people's fear, anxiety and so on.

- A pattern of lying, stealing, using aliases and law breaking.
- Frequent violation of the rights of others, unprovoked aggression or violence, imprudent or unsafe actions.
- Impulsiveness and irresponsibility.
- Lack of remorse after the performance of any of the above.

Here we could speculate that shame—an inhibitor—is being mistaken for anger—a driver of aggressive responses to people who cheat in performing social obligations. The biological function of anger in social animals is to punish cheaters. But in this situation, aggression arises in circumstances where restraint is appropriate. Common examples of a need for restraint include seeing that someone else is sad, fearful, anxious or nervous. Normally, we take such emotions in another person as a cue for restraint in our approach towards them—the effect of an inhibiting emotion, which makes us gentle with people who are suffering. People with antisocial personality disorder appear to be blind to this cue and the explanation that I offer here is that they interpret this inhibitor as anger.

PSYCHOPATHIC PERSONALITY DISORDER

Psychiatry has historically classified disorders based upon the symptoms, and in the case of antisocial personality disorder, the symptom is inappropriate aggression. However, anger is not the only emotion that drives aggression. The other major example is humiliation that drives males to retaliate against threats to biological fitness. This is likely to be a more violent form of aggression, but a classification based upon a symptom would just see it as a more extreme form of the same thing. Now that we can see that the emotions being mistaken for shame—anger and humiliation—are different, we should recognise that psychopathic and antisocial personality disorder are distinct. This distinction becomes important when we attempt to derive therapies for the treatment of such disorders.

Previously, in this section under Proactive Impulsion, when describing this structure I suggested that psychopathy resulted from misidentifying shame as humiliation resulting in inappropriate revenge responses, including to imagined threats. Psychopathy is heavily gender biased towards men,[116] which is what we would expect if the emotion of humiliation were a component of the cause.

BORDERLINE PERSONALITY DISORDER

This is perhaps the most widely studied acute personality disorder. The World Health Organization classification under ICD-10 for this condition is 'emotionally unstable personality disorder', which maybe captures its essence better.

- Impulsive and risky behaviour, such as changing homes or quitting jobs with only slight provocation, reckless sex, gambling or binge eating.
- Volatile and fragile self-image.
- Intense relationships that are unstable and transient—unreasonable fear of abandonment.
- Volatile mood, including anger, especially in response to stress. Since this is often caused by the condition itself, it leads to spiralling consequences.
- Self-harm including cutting or suicide, and threats to perform these actions.

In the case of borderline personality disorder, it appears clear that actions result from situations that normally require restraint. This fits the model of Proactive Impulsion, but it is difficult to determine what driving emotion they are mistakenly identifying. One possible explanation is that they are mistaking shame, a biological inhibitor, for anxiety, leading to panic responses in situations requiring restraint.

NARCISSISTIC PERSONALITY DISORDER

The principal symptoms of this disorder are:

- Affecting high social status, boastfulness, making dishonest claims about one's achievements in life and an exaggerated sense of entitlement.
- An assumption that others will or should admire you.
- Unreasonable and antisocial denigration of others as a means of maintaining an illusion of having a higher social status than them.
- A belief in high social status can lead to problems with over-consumption, over-spending and substance abuse.
- Although these symptoms appear superficially to be evidence of confidence, people with this condition respond to criticism or not getting their own way with rage, petulance and retaliation.

Narcissistic personality disorder, like psychopathy, is heavily male biased. This gives a clear clue that humiliation is involved, since this is the most notable example of a heavily male biased emotion. I believe that narcissistic personality disorder is a Deviant Proaction where a driving emotion is mistaken for humiliation. I cannot be certain which driving emotion is being misidentified and it is possible that different ones could give rise to very similar outcomes. Humiliation is an emotion that drives revenge responses against sources of threats to male biological fitness.

Let us suppose that a boy, during his formative years, experienced humiliation and another driving emotion, but he had been trained to suppress the behaviour associated with both. He was therefore unable to identify these emotions in himself. At some point, the other driving emotion arose and he incorrectly guessed that it was humiliation. Now, we have a set of circumstances that the boy (now grown into a man) incorrectly thinks will give rise to humiliation. But he is thinking proactively—he is trying to strategise future emotional outcomes. Clearly he is seeking to avoid future humiliation when he predicts a future occurrence of that circumstance that he incorrectly believes causes him humiliation. And the best way to achieve this is to pretend to be a male of high social status or, as a biologist would say, of high biological fitness.

This leaves an important question: why is it that mistaking an *inhibiting* emotion for humiliation gives rise to inappropriate violent revenge responses—psychopathy, whereas mistaking a *driving* emotion for humiliation gives rise to merely affecting high social status without the violence—narcissism? In the chapter Action Drivers and Action Inhibitors, I explained that with drivers, humans invert the causality of an action. For example, rather than hunger driving us to seek food, we understand future hunger so we seek food in advance to strategise the avoidance of that hunger. Pretending to be of high social status is an effective way of strategising the avoidance of future humiliation, and we can often observe this in males of low social status when they affect macho behaviour in their social interactions with one another. But proactive violence, in anticipation of imminent humiliation, is not an appropriate strategy to avoid it. With inhibiting emotions, it works differently. An inhibitor, like shame, causes the *non*-action state of *not* performing antisocial actions, but if an understanding of future shame causes us to strategise the non-performance of actions to avoid the future state of shame, this is the same thing as not performing the action in the present. I therefore speculate, that when a psychopath mistakes shame for humiliation, it is a misidentification that takes place in the present and so the response is the same as present humiliation, namely violent retaliation. This is different from strategising the avoidance of anticipated future humiliation. When men with narcissistic personality disorder are thwarted, criticised or slighted, they respond with rage and aggression—namely the symptoms of someone with antisocial or psychopathic personality disorder. I propose that this arises because this is mistakenly perceived as *present* humiliation and so prompts the action that biological humiliation is supposed to drive. Psychiatrists generally consider that narcissistic personality disorder has high comorbidity with antisocial and psychopathic personality disorders. In non-medical parlance, the two often occur together. But I suggest that a man of low social status is frequently criticised or slighted, so if he has narcissistic personality disorder this will regularly give rise to symptoms that converge with those of the other two personality disorders. This is not comorbidity, but a single condition.

HISTRIONIC PERSONALITY DISORDER

Histrionic personality disorder is a condition characterised by patterns of exuberant attention seeking. The symptoms include:

- Constantly seeking attention and discomfort when it is not obtained: self-dramatisation, theatricality, extravert and overly emotional.
- Inappropriately flirtatious and provocatively sexual.
- Obsessed with physical appearance as a means of obtaining attention.
- Shallow and constantly shifting emotions.
- Believes that relationships are more intimate than they actually are.
- Easily influenced and manipulated.

I believe that these symptoms correspond to a Deviant Proaction caused by someone mistaking a driving emotion for loneliness. Someone who is making this error of emotional identity will mistakenly predict future loneliness in certain circumstances. They will rationally deduce that they need to adopt a strategy to avoid this loneliness and so they will act in such a way as to attract the company of others.

Clearly, there is a question of which driving emotion is being mistaken. We need to consider that there are many more driving emotions than inhibiting ones. When we are confusing an inhibiting emotion, shame is most likely to be the one about which confusion arises. Looking at driving emotions, it may be possible to be confused about the identity of anger, jealousy, humiliation, guilt, loneliness, anxiety or revulsion—that is seven possibilities. If we assume that these are the only possibilities, then there are theoretically seven Deviant Anti-Impulsions, seven Proactive Impulsions, but 42 possible Deviant Proactions. (Each of the seven driving emotions listed above could be confused for any one of the other six driving emotions.) This is almost certainly an overestimate because it would appear unlikely that someone could confuse (for example) revulsion for loneliness or vice versa, but it does mean that Deviant Proaction is certain to be the structure with the most numerous potential outcomes. However, to give rise to a Deviant Proaction, we need someone to anticipate a future driving emotion where they are mistaken about the identity of that driver. This will cause them to proactively seek to manipulate that emotional outcome. I believe that the identity of the driver that they think it is has a bigger impact upon the outcome than the identity of the emotion that they are misidentifying. Therefore, which emotion they are mistaking as loneliness may not make that much difference.

It appears that the psychiatric profession is losing interest in histrionic personality disorder. It is certainly the case that there is little current research into this condition and there are predictions that it will soon disappear from both DSM and ICD in future editions.[117] It could be argued that this diagnosis, one of the only acute personality disorders with a heavy female bias, is the last remnant of a rather sexist historic approach in the development of psychiatry, where 'hysteria' was seen as an exclusively woman's madness.

CLUSTER C PERSONALITY DISORDERS

Psychiatrists call Cluster C personality disorders, the anxious, fearful cluster, and it would appear that each of these instances involves the emotions of anxiety or fear. Two of the Cluster C personality disorders, dependent and obsessive-compulsive, appear to fit the Deviant Proaction model, but avoidant personality disorder seems to fit the Deviant Anti-Impulsion model.

AVOIDANT PERSONALITY DISORDER

I believe that this acute personality disorder results from misidentifying anxiety with shame (i.e. the opposite error to what I suggested might cause borderline personality disorder). That makes it a Deviant Anti-Impulsion. The symptoms include:

- Avoidance of social situations for fear of being criticised or rejected.
- Avoiding starting projects for fear of failure.
- Feeling inadequate, inferior or unattractive.
- Fear of meeting new people, extreme shyness in social situations and personal relationships.
- Fear of disapproval, embarrassment or ridicule.

Anxiety is natural when meeting new people or starting new projects. Anxiety is what I call a strategic emotion—it encourages you to plan and prepare for hypothetical difficulties. It is probable that this emotion is unique to humans, who are the only animal on this planet that can form a complex understanding of the abstract future or abstract other places. In a situation of meeting new people or starting new projects, it is an effective way of sharpening the mind before facing challenges. If this emotion is mistaken for shame, then it will cause an inappropriate inhibition that becomes a huge impediment to attempting anything new in life. Applying the model with these emotional variables would appear to fairly accurately predict the symptoms of this disorder.

DEPENDENT PERSONALITY DISORDER

The symptoms of this disorder include:

- Inability to make decisions without constant reassurance.
- Inability to take responsibility for basic life functions and prefers to defer to others.
- Fear of disagreeing with anyone because of fear of loss of emotional support.
- Immediately seeks new partner upon a relationship terminating.
- Feels helpless when alone.
- Tolerance of abusive relationships due to a fear that the alternative is to be alone. Abuse is seen as the price of nurture or support.
- Unreasonable fear of being left alone.

One explanation of this situation could be that the person is mistaking anxiety, fear or loneliness for guilt. Guilt is a driving emotion that causes us to perform onerous social obligations. If we are mistaking another driving emotion for guilt, then we will incorrectly deduce the expectation of future guilt in unusual circumstances. The strategy for the avoidance of future guilt is attending to the observance of social obligation, perhaps in advance of the social obligation arising. A person with dependent personality disorder appears to be excessively attendant to their social obligations to family and romantic partners. They appear to live in fear of such people being disappointed in them, criticising them or being let down by them.

OBSESSIVE-COMPULSIVE PERSONALITY DISORDER

The last acute personality disorder in this cluster, obsessive-compulsive disorder, appears to involve misidentifying another driving emotion as fear or anxiety. However, I am reluctant to suggest which driving emotion is being confused. It is possible that confusing a number of different driving emotions as anxiety could have a similar outcome, but I do believe that this acute personality disorder is a Deviant Proaction. The symptoms include:

- Obsessive and unreasonable perfectionism in performing tasks.
- Inability to complete tasks, leading to distress, because the required standard is unobtainable.
- Inability to delegate because others will not tackle the task to the required standard of perfection.
- Neglect of relationships and enjoyable activities due to obsession with work functions.
- Narrow-minded morality and obsessive rule following in social relations.
- Rigid, stubborn and miserly.

If a person misidentifies another driving emotion as anxiety, then when they predict the circumstances that are the Biological Stimulus for that other emotion, they incorrectly deduce that they will experience future anxiety. The rational stategy is to seek to avoid that supposed future anxiety by an unreasonable level of over-preparedness for the avoidance of all possible misfortunes. This is the root cause of the perfectionist workaholism.

Most of us will want to have sufficient money in our bank account to cover expenditure for about a month or so, but for a person with obsessive-compulsive personality disorder they will predict future anxiety in unreasonable circumstances and will not feel secure unless they have sufficient money to cover expenditure for the year. This is the root cause of miserliness and hoarding. I also speculate that the root cause of the rules following petty morality and overformality in social relations springs from a misidentified anxiety of causing offence or being criticised.

RECLASSIFICATION OF ACUTE PERSONALITY DISORDER

Throughout this book, I have been somewhat critical of the approach in psychiatry for classifying illnesses without coming up with explanations for them. However, now that I am offering an explanation, I think that a reclassification is due.

TABLE 7: RECLASSIFICATION OF ACUTE PERSONALITY DISORDER

Deviant Proaction			
Personality Disorder	APA Cluster	This Driver is Misidentified . . .	. . . as this Driver
Narcissistic	B	Any driver*	Humiliation
Histrionic	B	Any driver*	Loneliness
Dependent	C	Anxiety, fear or loneliness	Guilt
Obsessive-compulsive	C	Any driver*	Anxiety
Proactive Impulsion			
Personality Disorder	APA Cluster	This Inhibitor is Misidentified . . .	. . . as this Driver
Antisocial	B	Shame	Anger
Psychopathic	Not APA recognised	Shame	Humiliation
Borderline	B	Shame	Anxiety
Deviant Anti-Impulsion			
Personality Disorder	APA Cluster	This Driver is Misidentified . . .	. . . as this Inhibitor
Paranoid	A	Humiliation	Shame
Schizoid	A	Loneliness	Shame
Avoidant	C	Anxiety	Shame

* I suggest that it does not matter which driver is being misidentified. What matters is what it is being misidentified *as*.

To summarise, Table 7 is how I would reorder acute personality disorders with the misidentification of emotions that lies at their origin.

This classification leaves out schizotypal personality disorder, in common with the current ICD-10 classification. Partly, I admit, I am leaving it out because I cannot make it fit into the model that I have described here.

D:
DELUSIONS

Love is merely a madness; and, I tell you,
deserves as well a dark house and a whip as
madmen do; and the reason why they are not
so punish'd and cured is that the lunacy is so
ordinary that the whippers are in love too.
— William Shakespeare, As You Like It

THE BRAIN AS A SELF-REFERENCING MECHANISM

When I lived in Brooklyn, the shoreline of New York Harbour had huge granite boulders that had been put there to prevent tidal erosion. Whenever I got bored (i.e. most days) I would walk to the harbour and jump from boulder to boulder until I was at the water's edge. Once, when I was doing this, I imagined slipping and falling between the rocks, and a numb sensation spread through my legs. I have noticed this happen on several occasions and it can sometimes occur when I think of someone else having an experience that would result in serious leg injury. For example, it once occurred when I was in the park and a small child painfully fell off her bike.

I became so intrigued by this phenomenon that eventually I started asking all my friends who were neuroscientists, neurologists and psychologists exactly what they thought was happening. Their answers were inconsistent, but our understanding of brain functionality is still somewhat embryonic. We know a vast amount, but the sheer complexity of a human brain means that what we do understand is still a fairly low percentage of the totality. That being said, we do know that the brain has several ways of registering pain, and once registered there are different responses to it. The most likely explanation of my numb feeling is that my brain released endorphins; this is an abbreviation of 'endogenous morphine', a form of opioid that exists naturally in the brain. It is released in certain situations of extreme exertion or threat and has an analgesic effect: it neutralises the sensation of pain. This is a brain routine kicking-in that has the purpose of managing pain, and the effect is that my legs felt numb. I am not particularly interested in researching long theses on the neuroscience stuff because I am going to follow a completely different line of enquiry.

What interests me is that an act of pure imagination can trigger an alteration in my brain state. The alteration in my brain state is supposed to be a reaction to real external events, such as *actually* breaking my leg or being chased by predators. If a pretended event that exists only in my imagination can cause these changes, then that means that a human brain can do something that a chimpanzee brain almost certainly cannot do. A chimpanzee does not have language and that limits its ability to form concepts. That in turn limits its ability to think in hypotheticals. It would be a fairly conventional view for both philosophers and animal behavioural scientists to suppose that a chimpanzee cannot speculate about a predator that is not actually there or a traumatic leg injury that has not actually happened. However, we all have to admit a certain level of philosophical doubt about this. Again, it would be a conventional view to suggest that a chimpanzee cannot think about thinking—this is an advanced cognitive capability that probably only exists in humans, but we cannot be completely sure. Thinking about thinking is so common in humans that we do not think about it much. Sorry! That was not supposed to be a joke, but in a '*cogito ergo sum*' sort of way, the mere fact that I can *talk* about thinking, implies that I can *think* about thinking. When you experience self-doubt, e.g. you consider whether you are capable of doing something or not, you are thinking about thinking. When you wonder why you keep imagining something that you would prefer not to imagine—again that is thinking about thinking. You can remember remembering something, even when you have forgotten what it was that you remember remembering.

There is another example of pure imagination triggering a brain reflex that only male readers will relate to, but there may be a female equivalent that I do not know about. When I imagine being kicked in the groin or I see this happen to another man, it can trigger the strange reflex where my testicles retract into my abdomen. With this situation and the thought of falling between the rocks there is an odd distinction that I have noticed. If I make a proactive decision to summon the imaginative image, my brain knows that it is an act of imagination and so the brain reflex does not occur. When my brain does not know this, in other words when the idea occurs to me as a result of some spontaneous thought or trigger, then my brain does not expect it and so the reaction occurs. I then started to wonder whether it would be possible to train myself, through meditation or otherwise, to summon the brain response at will. Yogis seem to have a strange talent for doing just this but, although I practise yoga, I am not sure that I want to take it to such extremes. However, towards the end of Section B: Compulsions, I explained that I trained myself to become depressed, which most people (even yogis) would consider to be highly abnormal. However, there is a curious example of this: when we imagine acts of sex or sexual situations, we become sexually aroused—the mere act of imagination causes a change in brain state and most of us can perform this at will (and sometimes against our will). Most of us have trained ourselves to think about sex without getting aroused. This avoids embarrassment when we think about it in a public place.

A human is a self-referencing mechanism. Computer scientists understand that self-referencing is the origin of circular causality. If you write '=A1' in cell A1 of a spreadsheet, then the memory cell self-references. The self-reference prevents the cell from computing any meaningful answer and the spreadsheet would be considered to have a circular argument. In old-skool computer programming language we write sequential lines of code. If at line 42, we tell the programme to go back to line 41, then the programme (rather than the memory cell) self-references. Unless the code at line 41 sends it somewhere else the programme will keep repeating lines 41 and 42 until someone pulls the plug out. Self-referencing is a pre-requisite of circular causality, and I have been focusing on the fact that humans self-reference in a way that has no equivalent in any other system that I can think of: we impersonate our own behaviour. Neither chimpanzees nor computers can do this. My work is mostly about exploring the consequences of this self-reference. When a human does this, it has consequences that could include circular causality, and this is in fact the origin of all forms of conceptual belief, whether religious, cultural or ideological. The models of compulsive action that we explored in Section B: Compulsions, all involve feedback loops that never switch off—an unusual consequence of the corruption of a biological system that is supposed to promote survival. Until we understand all the possible causal pathways that this self-referencing might drive, we will never understand ourselves.

If an act of pure imagination—in other words something that occurs in my brain—can trigger a change in a brain state—something else within my brain—that is supposed to be a reaction to something in the external world, then this is a self-referencing mechanism of an entirely different nature. What causal pathway could this set off? The one thing that is fairly certain is that these are pathways that are not the product of an animal that is a 'survival machine' in the shorthand of evolutionary theorists. It is a pathway that is more appropriate to a 'machine that is goal-seeking emotional outcomes', since I have now stumbled upon a way that I can change my emotional states by acts of pure imagination. I speculate that this could lead to hypothetical explanations of rational actions that would be recognised by psychiatrists as being mental disorders.

Psychiatry makes distinctions between neurosis, acute personality disorder and psychosis. These distinctions have been recognised since the nineteenth century, although more recently psychiatry has stopped using the term 'neurosis'. The logical structures that we constructed in Section B: Compulsions would fall into the category of neuroses and those in Section C: Impulsions would fall into the category of acute personality disorder—what I would simply call a rationally derived self-destructive action of a compound nature. A psychosis is something beyond this—a state where somebody appears to have completely lost touch with reality. A 'delusion' means more or less the same thing to a psychiatrist as it means to a layperson: a belief that is wildly different from observed reality.

People who hold such beliefs would normally be diagnosed as psychotic, but although they claim to hold crazy beliefs, there is a philosophical question (since there is no scientific way to analyse it) as to the nature of these beliefs. Evangelical Christians often claim that every word of the bible is literally true—a form of absolute belief that is frequently contradicted by observable reality. Hindus, by contrast, do not seem to have a problem with seeing the elephant god Ganapati as something allegorical—in other words you are not actually supposed to believe it, but you are still a Hindu. There is a subtle linguistic distinction here that religious critics tend to overlook: people *practice* Eastern religions, they do not *believe in* them. I often joke about being the world's only nihilist yogi: I practice yoga without believing in anything. Comparisons have been made (e.g. by Harris[118]) between madness and religion. I do not think these comparisons are helpful, but I am seeking to demonstrate that both have a logical structure. Despite this, the psychiatric profession remains vulnerable to a criticism of unsustainable inconsistency: if millions of us hold delusional beliefs, we call it a religion, but if one of us does, we call it a psychosis. We can take this further—religious fundamentalism is a delusional state where you believe you are practicing a religion, but actually your beliefs are something entirely different. I doubt that psychiatrists have any views on how we should explain or tackle that. Pinel, who was very influential in the development of early concepts of psychiatry, recognised 'religious madness' as a condition.[119] Perhaps he was the first to acknowledge the condition of religious fundamentalism. The difference between imagining something and believing it is quite subtle. It is clear that the writer J. R. R. Tolkien did not believe in Middle-earth, although *The Lord of the Rings* is clearly allegorical since it was inspired by the horrors of Nazism and World War II. It is not entirely clear whether a Hindu believes in Ganapati or that an evangelical Christian *really* believes every word. What I am suggesting is that if an act of imagination can trigger a change in a brain state, then this is a form of self-reference that opens up a world of possibility for emotional gratification. If we assume a human is a totally rational actor that is a machine that goal-seeks emotional outcomes, then how can a human think that he is the Pharaoh Sekhemresewadjtawy Sobekhotep III, or that he is being pursued by hideous monkey demons? Can we construct a hypothetical situation where thinking this is an entirely reasonable thing to do?

INTENTIONAL DELUSIONS

Scientists have tried practically every possible avenue in their attempt to figure out psychosis. Discovering how one works seems like a hopeless dream if we cannot even figure out what it is beyond a collection of symptoms. Research has focused on neuroscience, psychology, genetics and sociology, with recent efforts mostly concentrating in neuroscience. I am not a specialist in these technical fields, so I am not going to give you a long thesis that you could better obtain elsewhere. However, my project is to construct a hypothesis of how humans function based upon the assumption that they are logical computational devices. In a sense, neuroscientific knowledge is not a prerequisite of my project.

Although scientists are generally mystified by psychosis, they have understood for a while that the brains of schizophrenics have abnormally high levels of the neurotransmitter dopamine.[120] The same is true of people with bipolar disorder when they are in a manic phase. As every scientist knows, correlation is not causation, except that it almost always is, but we cannot deduce in which direction the causality travels. It is also possible that the schizophrenia and the high level of dopamine are both caused by a third something that nobody has yet discovered. Little scientific consensus has emerged, and nothing that looks like a description of a causal mechanism. All we can do is speculate. And that is what I propose to do as well. Since I am not a neuroscientist, I will reorient the dopamine hypothesis of schizophrenia to frame it as a philosophical problem, as opposed to a scientific one. The aim of this chapter is not to *explain* schizophrenia—that would be too grandiose a project—but merely to demonstrate that it can be rational to be delusional. It just so happens that the development of this idea arrives at a place that looks a lot like schizophrenia, but this might be the genesis of an idea that could apply to other forms of psychosis, and might well link to neurotransmitters other than dopamine—particularly serotonin. Therefore, I am going to describe it in a generic way to avoid the risk of either neuroscientific or psychiatric errors. This hypothesis could also apply to other delusions that link to other regulatory brain mechanisms that do not deploy neurotransmitters.

Firstly, we need to establish what a neurotransmitter is *for*. This question is different, in subtle ways, to establishing what they *do*. At some point in our evolutionary history, the genes that gave rise to a particular neurotransmitter function arose, and they were only selected because they enhanced the survival of the animal that carried them. If we can figure out how they enhanced survival, then we can understand what the neurotransmitter function is *for*. This question is hardly made any easier by the fact that dopamine can be found in earthworms and figuring out what it does for them is unlikely to help us understand what it does for schizophrenics. That is why it is important to consider the neurotransmitter *function* as it operates in an advanced vertebrate, rather than the chemical itself. There is a huge scientific literature on what they do, but I could not find anything on what they are for, so I set out to answer the question myself. I am adopting an adaptationist approach that is fairly normal for evolutionary theorists, so I might be recreating an explanation that has already been done before.[121]

Imagine you come home from a hard session at the gym. You are hungry, thirsty, tired and your skin feels icky, so you need to eat, drink, take a nap and have a shower. But before you can act, you need to decide the order in which to do those things. Hunger, thirst, tiredness and icky skin are emotions that drive actions, and each of them has an evolutionary origin: each feeling drives an action that enhances your survival. The evolutionary origin of the icky skin feeling may not be immediately obvious, but animals that do not attend to skin irritations get sores that ultimately kill them, so the icky feeling drives the animal to scratch or take a mud-bath to remove parasites. You have inherited the icky skin driver from your swamp-dwelling ancestors.

What happens when you get home from the gym is that these four feeling-based action drivers jostle against one another in your consciousness. Each of them is a thermostat that switches on a specific action routine. But they are not just on/off switches—they register a variable level that tells you how urgent it is that you undertake the action. Since each thermostat gives out a different reading, one will be highest and that achieves dominance and drives the action that you will perform first. Once you have attended to that (say you start with a drink, which will stop you being thirsty) the other three feelings will jostle against one another until you decide what is the next most important.

I am going to call this the 'Normal Mode' of interaction of different emotional action drivers, and why, will become apparent when I come to consider when it is ever necessary to vary from Normal Mode.

Putting on my mathematician's hat, it is not sufficient to take a static view of the relative strength of these four feeling-based action drivers. We also need to consider how they change according to how strong the need for action is. We could refer to this as the 'gradient', or what a mathematician would call the first derivative of the emotional action driver. Let us consider an example. Assuming that it can avoid exertion, a human can survive without food for up to two months, but it can only survive for about a week without water. We would therefore expect thirst to have a steeper gradient than hunger relative to the time since we last undertook the action that the feeling is supposed to drive. If we eat and drink to our full satisfaction and then do not attend to any of our bodily functions for a sustained period, we would expect our thirst to grow faster than our hunger so that when we are permitted to attend to our bodily functions, we would expect our thirst to be the dominant driver. That is to say that thirst would have a steeper gradient than hunger.

However, we should not expect the gradient (first order derivative in math speak) of each to be constant. We would expect the gradient to change too (what a mathematician would call the second order derivative). To optimise our chances of survival, we need to ensure that in every possible combination of relative thirst and hunger the right feeling emerges as the dominant driver, and therefore we would expect hunger and thirst to have a curve structure to ensure that this is the case.

I rather doubt that there is much written in the scientific literature about this. The reason for this is simple: the feeling that drives the action is a state of consciousness; scientists (like everyone else) have no idea what a state of consciousness is; and therefore, they do not have any way to measure a feeling. That is why it is impossible for a scientist to plot the curve structure of hunger, thirst or any other emotional action driver in a robust way, but they have attempted it. During World War II, American scientists performed experiments with volunteer conscientious objectors that became known as the Minnesota starvation experiment.[122] The scientists wanted to understand how to tackle the problems of starvation that they anticipated arising in Europe. The volunteer subjects of this experiment became obsessed with food and conserving energy, but the problem of how to plot the curve structure of hunger remained. One of the only situations in normal parlance where scientists pretend they can measure feelings is wind chill factor, but although there is no agreed method of working this out, it is generally computed by measuring the rate at which an inanimate object changes temperature as cold air moves around it. This is not a measure of feelings as such. When science cannot provide the answer, we have to turn to other sources, and the answers can be found in some surprising places.

Primo Levi was an Italian Jewish chemist who was sent to Auschwitz. He thought like a scientist, but wrote like Dostoevsky. During his time in Auschwitz, he was assigned work in sweltering heat without access to water for the duration of his shift. Levi compares in detail extremities of hunger and thirst that the rest of us are unlikely to experience. Extreme hunger, he says, is endurable; it is actually something to which you can become accustomed. But thirst is not endurable. It rapidly drives you to a state of crazy desperation. 'Hunger exhausts, thirst enrages.'[123] This would seem to imply that the curve structure of hunger is a slow climb to a level plateau; whereas thirst climbs rapidly, and may not hit a plateau before you fall into delirium. Thirst quickly emerges as the dominant action driver over hunger, and this is what we would expect as the outcome of evolution, since lack of water kills first. Let us consider the curve structure of another feeling-based action driver: pain. This drives the separate actions of recoiling from sources of injury and attending to a healing process. The curve structure of pain is that it switches on instantly and actually declines after an initial boost to a lower plateau. (It's those endorphins again!) It then does not switch off until the problem is resolved. Unlike hunger and thirst that drive us to resolve a problem that arises gradually, pain drives us to resolve a problem that arises instantaneously, and so we would expect it to rise and fall according to a different curve shape.

To consider what a neurotransmitter is for, I need to consider how they operate in animals. The danger of considering them in humans is that (as most of this project is devoted to explaining) we have language, and this permits us to tactically manipulate our expression of emotion and strategically seek emotional goals—we out-think our own biology. This is what leads to self-destructive actions. In short, language causes corruption of our emotions, and studying how they work in humans produces very confusing results. Let us therefore consider a lion that is hunting a zebra.

The lion and the zebra are in competition for a commodity: the zebra's body. Clearly, the lion and the zebra have different uses for this commodity and this has an impact upon how emotional action drivers will work for each of them. Firstly, we must recognise that the lion and zebra do not have equal and opposite interests. The lion does not care whether it eats this particular zebra's body or another, but the zebra cares very much about the lion's choice because it does not want to be eaten. The downside for the zebra of a successful hunt is infinite, but the upside for the lion is a finite quantity of nutrition. The downside of an unsuccessful hunt is equal and finite for both parties because of the energy wasted and the risk of injury. After an unsuccessful hunt both parties will need to rest and heal to prepare for the next encounter. Let us start by considering the variables from the point of view of the lion. It is easiest to visualise if we ascribe an approximated points system to what the lion is doing.

- If the lion catches the zebra, the food it gets is worth 50 points, but only half of hunts are successful.
- For every 100 metres that the lion has to run, the energy expended costs the lion 5 points, so in very simple terms, a lion should never consider chasing a zebra more than 500 metres. However, we have to adjust for the probability of the hunt being successful, so it should not attack unless it expects to run less than 250 metres, and the closer the lion is able to stalk before it attacks the better.
- The risk for the lion is getting kicked in the teeth, which prevents it from hunting and is therefore fatal. The Zebra can kick! Death is an infinitely negative outcome for the lion, but death also arises from not hunting, so the lion has to consider the relative probability of injury and hunt success. This permits us to score the probability-adjusted risk of injury. We can call this negative 1 point for the lion, which is mathematically equivalent to saying that (on average) a lion will receive a fatal injury on its one-hundredth hunt or fiftieth kill. (Note that, foolish though it might sound, the zebra on average receives a fatal injury on its first kill.)

So the lion has to consider three variables. Each of these variables is probabilistic. This would be simple if the lion could do mathematics. And since it cannot, evolution by natural selection has equipped the lion with a computational substitute. The lion has one emotional driver—hunger, and two emotional inhibitors—fear and tiredness. It is no coincidence that the inhibitors prevent outcomes that have negative scores in the above scheme, and the driver causes an outcome that has a positive score. Evolution by natural selection should shape each of these emotional action drivers/inhibitors into a curve. A lion where the gradient of the tiredness inhibitor is too steep will stop running too early in the hunt, and so it will die of starvation and with it the genes that caused its tiredness to become the dominant emotion in such an inappropriate situation. Evolution by natural selection will therefore shape the curves such that, with the lion operating in Normal Mode, in every possible situation the correct emotion emerges dominant.

Let us speculate about some of the ways that these three emotions might interact. All predators will occasionally tackle risky prey. For a lion, a buffalo is risky prey. Using the arbitrary scoring system we had earlier, let us say that a buffalo kill is worth 100 points (because it is twice the size of a zebra) and the probability of a hunt being successful remains at 50 per cent, and the energy involved in the hunt is double (because it takes two lions to bring down a buffalo) but the probability-adjusted risk of injury is worth minus 5 points for each of the lions involved in the kill. If this scoring system is correct, then lions should only hunt buffalos when there are no zebras, because the lions can achieve the same outcome by killing two zebras as one buffalo with less risk of injury. Again, with my mathematician's hat on, I can speculate about how evolution by natural selection could shape the curves of the emotional inhibitor that we normally call fear. The curve of this emotion should not be linear in proportion to the size of the prey. As the prey becomes bigger the fear curve needs to get steeper. This is because doubling the size of the prey does not double the probability-adjusted risk; it multiplies it by 5. (In math speak we need the second derivative of fear relative to size of prey to be positive.) Each of the feeling-based drivers of the lion will be shaped in such a way.

We now have a hypothetical mathematical model that explains why lions (acting in Normal Mode) do not hunt gazelles because the probability of the hunt being successful is too low, and why cheetahs do not hunt zebras (despite certainty of catching every one they chase) because the risk of injury is too high. The lions and cheetahs cannot work out the probabilities that should determine what they hunt, but they do not need to because their individual emotions of fear, hunger and tiredness have different shaped curves that result in each chasing the appropriate prey. Cheetahs just need to have a shallower tiredness curve, and a steeper fear curve with respect to size of prey. In every circumstance, for each species, the correct emotion becomes dominant in each situation. We now have a hypothetical mathematical model that explains why the lion has an 'instinct' to hunt zebras and the cheetah has an 'instinct' to hunt gazelles that is based entirely upon the mathematical function of three emotions. What else do they need other than teeth and claws?

Now let us apply the same methodology to the zebra. For the zebra, there is no upside to the hunt. Every 100 metres it runs costs it 5 points, but the cost of being caught can be considered to be infinitely negative. What then is the relevance of the cost of running? Tiredness is an emotional inhibitor that eventually stops the lion running, but it should never stop the zebra. Similarly, what is the relevance of the zebra being hungry or thirsty or in need of a scratch? Everything that the lion is doing can be seen in mathematical/probabilistic terms. But for the zebra, we need to disconnect Normal Mode. The zebra's actions need to be completely devoted to avoidance of a binary outcome. In theory, it should consider any cost as being worth paying. If the only way that the zebra can escape is to crash through thorny undergrowth, it should do this, but the lion should not follow because of the possibility of a fatal thorn in the paw. The lion is operating in probabilistic Normal Mode, but the zebra is not. The lion is pursuing a finite upside, but the zebra is fleeing an infinite downside. So what is the relevance of the curve shape of the zebra's tiredness inhibitor? In fact, there is only one driver that matters, and that is fear. However, a strange inversion has occurred that, upon reflection, is completely obvious. Fear is an emotional inhibitor for the lion, but for the zebra it is a driver. One way of looking at this is that a predator has an instinct to run towards danger and prey has an instinct to run away from it.

But if we consider the mathematical values that we have ascribed to this situation, fear in the lion prevents a negative outcome by stopping the lion tackling the most risky prey, and it prevents a negative outcome in the zebra by making it run away faster. Either way, the shape of the mathematical curve of fear as a driver of the zebra is irrelevant since it is driving an action that prevents a binary outcome. It therefore must dominate over all other emotions until the danger has passed, and the simplest way to achieve this is switch all the others off. When a zebra is fleeing from a lion, tiredness should never be an inhibitor, nor should the pain of injury slow it down. So we have now arrived at a hypothesis for what dopamine release and its effect on the appropriate receptor is *for*. It switches an animal (that cannot do mathematics) from a probabilistic Normal Mode of operation driven by the interplay of multiple emotions, to a binary mode of operation driven by a single one. To understand neurotransmitters, we need to stop thinking of them as a chemical, and start thinking of them as a mathematical function. They are binary disconnectors of emotional drivers and inhibitors that are themselves mathematical formulae: a curve representing the relationship between a particular biological need and the urgency of acting to rectify it.

Fleeing lions is not the only situation where such a situation arises. If we stopped sex when we got tired, then none of us would have offspring. Neuroscientists often claim that dopamine is somehow connected to the brain's reward system, but it could be that what we think of as a positive emotional outcome is actually the effect of all our emotional inhibitors being switched off for a moment. The ecstasy of sex could actually result from all emotional inhibitors being disconnected. This is a pretty good starting hypothesis for explaining a lot of human sexual activity that is very regrettable the next morning. Sex tends to cause the brain to produce endorphins too, so that you are insensitive to pain—a dry martini of neurotransmitters. (Shaken, presumably, not stirred!)

Let us switch back to humans (that can do mathematics). I will take off my mathematician's hat and put on my philosopher's hat because I now have to concern myself with the imposition of language into this process.

We have already considered how you determine the order of satisfying your bodily needs when you come home from the gym. So it would appear that in Normal Mode, you operate in much the same way as the lion. But when does a human leave Normal Mode? When the neurotransmitters that were released in the hunted zebra are released in your brain, will you operate in the same way as the zebra? This is a bit difficult to determine because we cannot ethically put humans into near-death situations in a laboratory. However, World War I veterans that actually survived often recalled that 'going over the top', or in other words leaving the safety of their trench and walking towards rattling machine guns, caused a sensation of intense elation—circumstances of extreme threat caused the neurotransmitter release that switched off all negative emotional experience. We have other examples from the battlefield: there are anecdotes of soldiers who were caught in vicious fire-fights who only realised that they had been shot when it was all over—in other words, in a near-death moment similar to the hunted zebra, their brain released the neurotransmitter that temporarily switched-off all awareness of pain. This makes perfect sense.

So, if this is all exactly as it is supposed to be—precisely how evolution by natural selection has optimised our chances of survival—can the process go wrong in a human in a way that cannot happen in a zebra?

My work is devoted to demonstrating that a human is a robustly logical computational device that goal-seeks emotional outcomes, and we are now contemplating whether this might still be true of someone who thinks he is pursued by fire-breathing fishwives with glinting trident spears, when actually he is strapped to a bed in a mental hospital. Logic is a function of language—something that only humans have. Language permits us to form concepts—something that only humans can do. It permits us to form concepts of emotion and behaviour and we have evolved (that is culturally, not by natural selection) to tactically alter the projection of our emotional behaviour and to strategise the achievement of emotional goals. What I have been explaining is that this process corrupts the action drivers and inhibitors that evolution by natural selection provided to us. Our lives become dominated by the aim to achieve emotional goals, and manipulating our emotional behaviour alters our perception of those goals and creates beliefs that ultimately are nothing other than theories about how to achieve emotional goals. So if we twist the emotions that evolution by natural selection gave to us, do we inadvertently (or intentionally) twist the operation of our neurotransmitters?

Absolutely we do! Let us consider some examples:

Situation 1: you go on a rollercoaster. This simulates a near-death experience (safely) and tricks your brain into thinking you are in a similar situation to the hunted zebra. Your brain releases a dopamine rush that produces a feeling of complete euphoria. We think of this as a positive emotional experience (which it is) but the neuro-electronics of it likely have more to do with the switching off of all emotions that we associate with negative experiences. It is actually quite hard, to come up with an evolutionary explanation of the existence of a positive emotion.

Situation 2: you self-medicate drugs (preferably very illegal ones). There are two ways of increasing dopamine concentrations in the forebrain: one is to increase its release, and the other is to slow down its reuptake (since the brain constantly releases small quantities of dopamine). Amphetamines, cocaine, some opiates, nicotine, phencyclidine and cannabis all increase dopamine levels by one of other of these two methods.[124] This produces a similar experience to going on a rollercoaster—an experience of total aliveness. Again, you are seeking emotional outcomes by manipulating the neurotransmitter state of your brain. Amphetamines actually produce similar symptoms to paranoid schizophrenia.[125]

Situations 1 and 2 are examples of humans strategically seeking emotional goals that involve the manipulation of neurotransmitters by external means. But can we manipulate them without external means? Yes we can!

Situation 3: soldiers are taught that when they come under fire, the first thing to do is hit the ground; the second is to roll to cover; and the third is to control their breathing. As soon as they have found cover, they take slow deep breaths. This has the effect of persuading the brain that everything is perfectly normal. By adopting a behavioural technique they can cause their brain *not* to release the dopamine. If they did not do this and the dopamine was released, they would hyperventilate and the only thing they would be good for would be running away.

Situation 4: on the starting blocks of the 100 metres Olympic final, a sprinter 'psyches himself up'. What exactly is involved with this process? Is it possible that a human can do something that an animal cannot do? By an act of pure imagination, can we visualise ourselves in a situation of danger and thereby persuade the brain to release dopamine? If the sprinter could do this, then he would have no awareness of the tiredness in his muscles towards the end of the race.

Situations 1 and 2 demonstrate that we want to achieve dopamine release, and Situation 3 demonstrates that we can manipulate dopamine release by purely behavioural measures. However, Situation 3 achieves dopamine suppression, whereas what I want to demonstrate is that we can stimulate dopamine release without external means as in Situation 4.

The dopamine hypothesis of psychosis exists because the brains of people with schizophrenia and other psychoses have been found to have abnormally high levels of dopamine. This is a correlation, and correlation is not the same as causation. However, nobody understands the causation of psychosis and most named mental illnesses are little more than correlations of symptoms. But the dopamine hypothesis of psychosis seems to imply that dopamine somehow causes psychosis, and what I want to propose instead is that the causality is the other way round.

Let us say, for the sake of argument, somebody discovers that by enacting a particular behaviour pattern or by focusing their mind in an act of pure imagination, they can trick their brain into releasing dopamine without needing any external stimulus. Say for example, that they imagined being pursued by something hideous and screamed in horror at the thought. This particular behaviour pattern would likely appear rather weird to other people. In fact, they would probably think them mad! But why care about that? If you can trick your brain into the dopamine release, then you achieve a feeling of total aliveness as all negative emotions are switched-off. By doing this, you achieve an ecstatic state in which there is no consciousness of hunger, pain, tiredness or fear. You likely also lose all inhibitions regarding what others think of your behaviour, including psychiatrists!

Is that not something that somebody would actually want to do? In fact, once they have mastered the technique is it not something that they would do for all their waking hours?

A human with language can form concepts of abstract space and time that permit it to conceptualise its future. This gives humans the ability to plan that animals lack. In turn, this leads to the inversion of the causality of emotions. The actions of highly evolved animals like lions are driven by feelings. But human actions are driven by the desire to achieve emotional outcomes—in other words, we know that feelings are going to arise in the future, so we plan to prevent negative feelings arising and we strategise the achievement of positive ones. In non-speaking animals, emotions push actions, but in humans, actions pull emotions. Here, we have been exploring another possibility—that acts of pure imagination can also pull emotions. In fact, they can do so in ways that may well be more powerful than actions. But if an outcome of intense emotional elation can be achieved by combining actions and imagination in a way that triggers neurotransmitter release, then would it not be correct to say that pursuing that set of actions is entirely rational? It could therefore be the case that even psychotic delusions are compatible with my assumption that a human is a robustly logical computational device that goal-seeks emotional outcomes.

There are some strange supporting facts that suggest that this hypothesis is probably true. The first is that schizophrenics are known to have astonishing insensitivity to physical pain and extreme cold. This would fit in both with the hypothesis of what the neurotransmitter actually does and why a psychotic person strategises its release. Secondly, the usual antipsychotic medications for psychoses such as schizophrenia are drugs that deactivate dopamine receptors (and occasionally serotonin receptors). There has been a huge amount of research into drugs that are dopamine antagonists— these are chemicals that compete with dopamine for dopamine receptor sites, but do not have the effect of dopamine at these sites.[126] These have the effect of a total 'cure', that is, they stop the symptoms happening without any theory as to what caused the symptoms in the first place. This would seem to be a fantastic outcome, but the problem is that each year approximately three quarters of people prescribed psychotropic medicines relapse because they refuse to take their medications.[127] If the model for psychosis that I have described here is correct, then if their greatest possible emotional fulfilment is achieved by engineering a neurotransmitter release by a set of actions and thoughts that other people consider madness, then this would make refusing your medications a rational thing to do; since we should expect that for a schizophrenic person, the 'cure' would seem like a total let-down.

A real cure would involve trying to find the source of the pain that the schizophrenic is trying to neutralise by doing a selfie with his own neurotransmitters. It is not surprising that this is such a challenge, since we are trying to discover this with a person who is deliberately creating myths about their own emotional experience. Some psychiatrists working with schizophrenics are trying to move away from antipsychotic medications back to cognitive behavioural therapy, but this is a slow process.[128] We still hardly know where to begin.

E:
CONSEQUENCES

The Head-shakers have a formal vocabulary
of their own, which, after a certain
experience, one begins to know by heart. It is
constructed on the simple principle of giving
a bad name to everything.
— Herman Charles Merivale, My Experiences
in a Lunatic Asylum by a Sane Patient

THE POOR, THE MAD AND THE CRIMINAL

Let private asylums, where it is in the interest of
the proprietors to keep the patients as long as
they can, be swept away.
— Herman Charles Merivale, My Experiences in
a Lunatic Asylum by a Sane Patient

A convenient place to get rid of
inconvenient people.
— Andrew Scull, The Victorian Lunatic Asylum[129]

How does a society dispose of its unwanted people? How does it define those people? Who decides?

Every age and culture has had its own paranoia about the classes of people that are perceived to be the cancer of society. In the medieval world, lepers were considered to be the nadir of undesirability, and they were herded into colonies to quarantine them. The reason for this was ignorance and fear about the causes of leprosy and its contagion. Mad people were often considered to be 'holy fools' and were left to wander and beg. Generally, they were seen as benign. Sometimes it was considered to be lucky to give them alms, and this belief still survives in parts of modern day India. But as leprosy subsided in Europe, the mad gradually took over their role at the bottom of the human pecking order. Madness came to be seen as an affliction, since the concept of mental illness had not yet arisen. Generally, the medieval man believed that God sent madness as punishment for moral failings. However, poverty often led to both crime and madness. Consequently, the boundary between poverty, madness and criminality was blurred. Constant twisting of the lens over the centuries has never bought these distinctions into focus.

In seventeenth century France, the king decreed that begging was to be banned in Paris and all beggars were to be swept up and placed in the *Hôpital Général*. This was not a policy dictated by the rule of law as we idealise it in modern democracies. It was driven by a need to perpetuate a sanitised vision of society as held by the powerful. When the king went out on his carriage rides, he only wanted to see beautiful people; so the unsightly portion of humanity was literally swept away. People were held under a document called a *'lettre de cachet'*, which was an order under the king's private seal to inter without trial anybody who fell foul of someone who had influence at court. The numbers caught up in this sweep are shocking. By 1662, the *Hôpital Général* gave food and lodging to around 6,000 people which, at the time, was approximately 1 per cent of the population of Paris.[130] The most famous person to be held under a *lettre de cachet* was Marquis de Sade. His mother-in-law instigated this in 1777 after he absconded with his seventeen-year-old sister-in-law. People at court were so shocked by this that it was decided he must be mad and interring him was an easy way of pretending that he did not exist. De Sade was so held until all such prisoners were released when the *ancien régime* came to an end with the French Revolution.[131]

This policy was so successful in cleaning up the city and making it a better place to live for anyone *not* so interred that, on 16 June 1676, the king issued a royal edict ordering the establishment of an *Hôpital Général* in every city of the kingdom. Some of these were created from decommissioned leper colonies. Foucault documents the enthusiasm with which this supposed noble cause was taken up:

> The Archbishop of Tours was proud to announce on 10 July 1676 that his 'metropolitan city had fortunately foreseen the wishes of the King and erected a *Hôpital Général* called *La Charité* before the Paris hospital had come into being, with an organisation which

has long been a model for all hospitals subsequently created, both within the kingdom and beyond.'[132]

The idea of setting up a hospital system appears to be incredibly enlightened for the seventeenth century, but let us not get blinded by the fact that they adopted propagandist names like *La Charité*. At the time, the concept of disease was not well understood and when it was there was not a cure. Consequently, diagnosis was a rather random, mystical process in which physicians were experts because they all collectively proclaimed themselves as such. Almost none of their 'expertise' was evidence-based. As Foucault puts it: 'Hospitalisation and internment were independent of medicine, but even within medicine itself, theory and therapy only communicate in an imperfect reciprocity.'[133] Poor people could not afford physicians and people interred in the *Hôpital Général* were given food (gruel) and lodging (a prison cell)—against their will or course—but nothing in the way of medical treatment. There was little distinction between the concept of illness and moral failing and, in any case, most of them were there because they had been found begging on the streets. If they were sick, they likely became that way because urban poverty eventually makes everybody sick. Otherwise, they would surely become sick shortly after their arrival on account of the appalling living conditions. Any sick person whose family could provide for them (no matter how modest the provision) was cared for at home. Thus, the concepts of poverty, moral fault and madness merged into one. Poor people were poor because of moral fault, and madness was a punishment sent by God for moral fault. But sending such people to a prison that was actually called a 'hospital' created a tidy false impression that society was benevolent and merciful.

The distinction between moral fault and madness has shifted subtly over the centuries. Until the end of the eighteenth century, it was generally believed that mental illnesses were the psychological effect of a moral fault. This, of course, meant that the mad did not need to be pitied, since their affliction was their own fault. Foucault illustrates this with a quote from François Leuret from 1834:

Do not use consolation, for it is useless. Do not use reasoning, for you will not persuade. Do not be sad with melancholics, as your sadness will confirm theirs; nor should you be gay with them, or they will feel offended. What is needed is a cool head, and whenever necessary, a dose of severity. Your reason should control their behaviour. The only string that still vibrates within them is pain; be courageous enough to pluck it.[134]

Into the nineteenth century there was a gradual shift away from punishment towards moral education as a therapy: 'Psychology, as a means of cure, was organised around the idea of punishment. Before seeking to soothe, it inserted suffering within the rigours of moral necessity.'[135] The great mental health reformers of the period, like Pinel and Tuke, sought to take the element of inhumane punishment out of the management of the mad, but still madness was seen as the result of moral failing. Rather than punishing for moral failings, they sought to teach through 'moral methods' that bought madness and its cure into the domain of guilt. Much of their therapy consisted of forcing the mad to admit to their guilt. Foucault also quotes Pinel from the beginning of the nineteenth century: 'How important it is, to prevent hypochondria, mania and melancholia, to follow the immutable laws of morality.'[136] However, the moral element of incarcerating the mad was also seen as an important deterrent to moral failings in society as a whole.

These guarded asylums ... are retreats as useful as they are necessary ... the appearance of these dark places and the guilty souls that they contain is ideal for warning licentious youths of the dangers of their ways; so much so that prudent fathers and mothers do well to ensure that their offspring are familiar with these awful, detestable places from an early age, showing them these places where shame and moral turpitude are attached to crime, and demonstrating that men who have soiled the essence of their being often lose forever the rights to which society had entitled them.[137]

The seemingly obvious problems of permitting the mad and the criminal to mingle in institutions took a while to emerge. Mirabeau argued:

> I might ask ... why libertines and rascals are mingled together ...
> I might also ask why young people with a dangerous disposition
> are left with men who will quickly lead them to the last degree of
> corruption ... if this mixing of rascals and libertines exists, as it all
> too clearly does, why then by this infamous, odious union do we
> convict ourselves of that most heinous of crimes, that of forcing
> men into criminality.[138]

These changing attitudes gradually led to new reforms that came about in recognition of the need to separate the mad from the criminal. Orders were made at the end of the eighteenth century to remove the mad to hospitals specially made for this purpose. However, these did not yet exist and still there was no idea about how to manage the mad over the long term. However, such reforms were the true beginning of positive psychiatry: the mad should not simply be confined, but should be seen as innocent sufferers and should be looked after humanely. Moreover, they were increasingly cared for by medical personnel. There was no question of the mad being permitted to mingle with society, so this gave birth to the asylum, and since there were still lingering ideas that the mad had to be educated morally, they were put to work for the profit of their keepers and society. New theories emerged that asylums should permit the mad to wander the grounds because a degree of confined liberty was therapeutic.

The separation of madness from criminality led to another development in that 'crimes of passion' came to be recognised. Foucault cites the first such legal defence strategy as occurring in France in 1783.[139] This was regarding the defence of a man who had killed his mistress after finding her and another man in flagrante delicto. Here it was argued that he had a momentary madness that was of the highest form of morality. His defence appealed to the violent urge in all of us to respond to an act of the most serious insult performed against us. Madness is now divided into 'bad madness' that we cannot envisage in ourselves, and 'good madness' that we can imagine being overtaken by ourselves when prompted by a given stimulus. From this, it followed that madness was no longer something to be feared, but something that existed in all of us. Forensic psychiatry became a driving force in the development of psychiatry as a science. Another such example is James Hadfield, who in 1799 tried to assassinate King George III, but his trial was halted when the defence convinced the judge that he had acted under an insane delusion.[140] It had long been a principle of law that the insane could not be punished for criminal acts. However, this was never a problem if they could be interred just as easily for madness as for criminality. In the nineteenth century, psychiatrists were frequently employed in criminal trials, and the principle became established that only they could tell if someone was truly insane. The insanity plea was applied with such diverse outcomes that eventually the English courts devised the M'Naghten Rules (1844) to create a legalistic formula that criminal trials could use as a guide.[141] These rules state (in summary) that a person is presumed sane until proven otherwise, and it must be demonstrated that he or she was so deluded that they had no way of knowing the nature of the act they were performing or that it was wrong. These rules, or variations on them, still have relevance in most common law jurisdictions, but they have always been controversial and have left plenty of room for confusion. For example, the idea of monomania started to arise in criminal trials: someone who was completely functional could have a single homicidal outburst for which they were not responsible due to a temporary madness.[142] This is a convenient ticket to get-out-of-jail free, since you are not criminally liable on account of insanity, but your insanity was temporary so there is no need to send you to an asylum. In general though, by the nineteenth century we arrived at a point where certain types of action resulted in your interment, and whether you were mad or not just determined whether the institution was a prison or an asylum. How you ran your legal defence would depend upon which happened to be the best outcome at the time.

The uncertainty of what constituted madness inevitably caused some horrific miscarriages of justice and created some great causes célèbres. Louisa Lowe was an Englishwoman who had been married to a clergyman for almost three decades. In 1870 she decided to leave him, and he arranged for her to be kidnapped and committed to a mental institution where she was trapped in a legal limbo for eighteen months. She was a wealthy woman, and while she was so conveniently indisposed, the private asylum owner and her husband asset-stripped her through bogus charges or application to the courts to seize her property. Upon her release, she founded the Lunacy Law Reform Association to campaign for the rights of people who became trapped in the asylum system—many of whom were sane.[143] A similar case in America was Clifford Whittingham Beers, a Yale graduate who was diagnosed with depression and paranoia that resulted in his internment in an asylum. He was released in 1903 after suffering horrific abuse and tyranny. In 1908, he wrote a book *A Mind that Found Itself*, and a year later he formed the Mental Hygiene Society.[144] This later became the Mental Health America—a campaigning organisation for the proper treatment of the mentally ill.

These campaigning organisations led to a shift away from asylums as places for incarcerating undesirables towards being places of cure. New asylums opened up that sought to only confine mad people for their own protection and for the purposes of imposing therapy. This would have been fabulous had a cure been found, but for the most part it has not—even today. Therefore, we are still facing the same problems that we faced centuries ago regarding how we should manage people whose self-destructiveness is compulsive or systematic or whose destructiveness of others does not fit neatly into the rules of society.

The problem of distinguishing between the mad and the criminal persists right to this day—complete with all the old controversies. Freud, in the first quarter of the twentieth century, normalised madness and made it something that we all had to some degree. He took away the stigma by persuading us that we all had a bit of it; so everybody could talk about it—including discussing their own 'complexes'. Criminality was the output of an unconscious mind that had somehow got the wrong stuff in it, but since we never knew what that stuff was it did not solve the problem. Szasz, since he believed that mental illness was a myth, inevitably became a fierce opponent of the idea that an insane person could not be criminally liable. 'Psychiatry rests on two profoundly immoral forensic practices: civil commitment and the insanity defence.'[145] But criminal law continues to have an input in psychiatry. In the 1950s, the criminal law first considered how to deal with psychopathy, which was described in English legal jargon as 'moral defectives of higher intelligence'.[146] But whereas a psychiatrist would regard psychopathy as a medical diagnosis within the spectrum of antisocial personality disorder, the dangers of managing such people means that prison is the only safe place for them. Therefore, even today concepts of madness are very different in law and medicine. Legal madness is based upon who gets harmed and medical madness is based upon whether the action was compulsive or uncontrolled. The problems of managing people who are compulsively destructive towards others, leads to a 'lock-em up and throw away the key' mindset, that is not a long-term solution either—effectively a return to the situation of centuries ago, where no distinction was made between madness and criminality.

Today, we have three ways of attempting to manage the mad: pills, talk therapy and incarceration. Surveys performed on treatments used show sharp divisions by socio-economic group.[147] Poor people with mental health problems tend to be prescribed pills (at least until they are jailed), and wealthy people get talk therapy. The reasons for this are clearly economic. Wealthy people seek treatment for their own benefit. They have better insurance or they can pay for it privately. Poor people do not have the means to pay for treatment. The emphasis is therefore that the government seeks to contain them in the cheapest possible way. This usually means pills rather than talk therapy.

We knew as early as the 1960s that persons with mental illness were disproportionately poor, but that their fathers were not.[148] These studies have been repeated in many countries.[149] This makes it pretty clear that mental illness causes poverty rather than the other way round. However, America is creeping back to the discredited incarceration policies of the eighteenth century. Then, we sent the mad to hospitals that were really prisons. Increasingly throughout the developed world, society makes very little provision to assist seriously mentally ill people, and if they are poor and cannot pay for assistance, it is inevitable that they will ultimately do something that is sufficient reason to lock them up; so we send them to a prison that has to fulfil the role of a hospital with almost none of the appropriate facilities. As one report put it: 'The most striking change in the care of persons with mental illness in the United States in the last three decades has been the transfer of responsibility from mental health professionals to law enforcement officers.'[150] The police are the de facto first responders when the mentally ill get themselves into difficulty, and they are therefore effectively an outpatient department without suitable training. This is not a failure of the criminal justice system. It is the combined effect of the failure of psychiatry as a project for managing people who cannot manage themselves, together with an unwillingness of government to fund proper care or research.

A report on the criminal justice system in New York City demonstrated that the city's prison population had declined 6 per cent in the period from 2005 to 2011, but the number of mentally ill people within the system had increased 26 per cent. The percentage of people in the prison system currently diagnosed as mentally ill has increased over this short period from 24 per cent to 33 per cent.[151] To put these numbers into context, the insanity plea is only used in 0.85 per cent of felony trials in America and the acquittal rate due to insanity is only 0.26 per cent.[152] Yet despite this lapse back into the abandoned policies of centuries past, the facilities for managing

them have barely improved at all. Inmates with acute mental illnesses like schizophrenia or bipolar disorder are 'supervised by
uniformed men and women who are often poorly trained to deal
with mental illness, and rely on pepper spray, take-down holds and
fists to subdue them.'[153] A report by The New York Times stated
that: 'Not since the gang riots of the 1980s and early 1990s has violence at Rikers Island so alarmed oversight officials, union leaders
and inmate advocates.'[154] Rikers Island is New York City's main
prison, and has seen the rate at which correction officers use violence
increase approximately five-fold in a decade. The title 'correction
officer' together with 'Department of Corrections' which is the official name of the American prison system itself denotes a rather
antiquated concept of moral instruction. Yet, the American prison
system invests very little in correction of antisocial behaviour and
encouraging rehabilitation.

Not only is this system confusing mental illness with criminality,
it is criminalising poverty. In some cases it is directly criminalising
homelessness.[155] The bail system is a mechanism for creating a financial incentive for people to show up for their court hearings. But the
poor cannot afford bail, so they wait in jail until their cases are
heard. In America, almost half a million people are in jail without
convictions awaiting trial.[156] That is 21.6 per cent of the total prison
population. A millionaire murderer can post bail and walk free,[157]
but a poor person awaiting a hearing on a misdemeanour charge
remains behind bars—effectively jailed for being poor.

To understand this problem further, it is necessary to go back to
1955, which was the year that America started a process of deinsti-
tutionalising mental health. At that time, the patient population of
mental hospitals in America was 558,239 out of a total population
of 164 million.[158] In other words, 0.34 per cent of the population
was a mental hospital inpatient. But shortly after that time, the
population steeply declined following a policy of closing mental
hospitals and treating their former patients in the community.
Often, this meant abandoning their treatment or significantly reduc-
ing it. The main catalyst for this policy was the introduction of

chlorpromazine (generally called Thorazine) that was the first effective antipsychotic medication. This led to a false optimism that the problem of mental illness could be solved with medicine. By 1994, the population of mental hospitals in America had fallen to 71,619, and after allowing for the increase in the population of the country, this accounted for a 91.3 per cent deinstitutionalisation.[159] Today, Rikers Island—a prison—holds more mentally ill people than all the mental hospitals in New York State combined. When people with mental health problems encounter problems with the police, there is nowhere left to care for them other than prison. This has led to the effective de-recognition of the insanity plea in criminal courts. Four states do not permit the insanity plea at all. Others officially use a form of the M'Naghten Rules or some variation of them. However, since there are no medical institutions for caring for violent or troublesome mental patients, the courts try to find ways around these. They apply tests, such as 'fit to stand trial', had 'the capacity to know right from wrong' or was 'capable of forming intent'. This often involves a court appointed psychiatrist claiming that they were simultaneously mentally ill and not insane[160]—a contradiction that is rarely scrutinised in court, since the objective of the court is to get such people off the streets where jail is the only available option. As Roy Porter explains it: 'Disputes over the insanity defence (who was bad? who was mad?) highlighted conflicts between legal and psychiatric models of the person, and left the public standing of psychiatry dubious.'[161] Some court appointed psychiatrists have a lucrative side income regularly telling the court what they want to hear. They would rarely be asked to opine on whether the M'Naghten Rules would indicate acquittal, since there is no alternative suitable institution for the management of people who cannot manage themselves. And to send them to prison, we need a criminal conviction. The effect of this is that mentally ill people gradually accumulate in prisons that are not equipped to deal with them. Between 25 and 40 per cent of mentally ill Americans will be jailed or incarcerated during their life.[162] A 2006 study found that more than half of the American prison population had a serious mental disorder compared to approximately 11 per cent of the general population that met DSM–IV criteria for a mental disorder.[163] This represents a population of over a million mentally ill people in American prisons out of a population of 300 million.[164]—almost exactly the same percentage as were mental hospital inpatients in 1955. But fewer than a third of these mentally ill prisoners receive psychiatric care.[165]

Sometimes psychiatric care is cynically withheld. A bipolar prisoner had his prescription of Seroquel terminated by the prison psychiatrist, who told him 'we don't give out feel-good drugs here'.[166] A prisoner in the same facility chewed off his finger, swallowed a toothbrush and cut open his abdomen to retrieve it, smashed open his own forehead and poured fluid into his brain, and cut open his scrotum to remove a testicle (among many other things). Yet the psychiatrist he was sent to by the prison determined that he was 'not in need of inpatient psychiatric treatment or psychotropic medication'.[167] This was in an American federal supermax prison, where many of the beds are equipped with strap-down rings like the mental hospitals of the nineteenth century. This is truly a regressive situation.

It is the thesis of this book that mental illness is in fact a series of logic problems that derive from mistaken ideas of emotion. If this view becomes accepted as correct, it ought to lead to a drift away from drug therapy back towards talk therapy as the most effective solution. Hopefully, that would eventually reduce the number of mentally ill people being housed in jails for want of a more suitable means of managing them. Clearly, my work would be more complete if I could suggest how such talk therapy would work. I cannot do this at present, but finding a solution to a problem must start with an accurate statement of the problem.

Consider the comparison between Anti-Compulsions and Libertine Compulsions. These are exactly the same mechanism, but in mirror image to one another. An Anti-Compulsion is a compulsion *not* to do something that you ought to do—like eating; and a Libertine Compulsion is a compulsion to do something that you ought *not* to do—like killing people. In most cases, anti-compulsives self-harm, so they are pitied and medicalised. Libertine compulsives usually cause harm to others; so they are vilified and criminalised. These are essentially the same mechanism and you do not get to choose your compulsive state. Our general ignorance of understanding the motivations of criminal acts, usually ends up with us stating that serial killing is a choice. Society judges you based on who you harm, not on why you do it. But few people think that anorexia nervosa—an Anti-Compulsion with respect to eating— is a choice. The idea that any compulsion is a choice is ridiculous, since if it were, it would not be a compulsion. Another absurdity is the idea that punishment is necessary to act as a deterrent to people to not perform criminal acts. A recent exponent of this view is Harris:

> If we made sneezing illegal, for instance, some number of people would break the law no matter how grave the consequences. A behaviour like kidnapping, however, seems to require conscious deliberation and sustained effort at every turn—hence it should admit of deterrence. If the threat of punishment could cause you to stop doing what you are doing, your behaviour falls squarely within conventional notions of free will and moral responsibility.[168]

And the threat of punishment only seems like a deterrent to people who would not perform the action anyway. Ask yourself how short the prison sentence for murder would have to be before you would consider killing someone who inconveniences you? In nature, intra-species killing is very rare and we have evolved mechanisms that prevent this. Threat of punishment has absolutely no impact on the likelihood that I will kidnap someone. If we assume that a serial killer has a Libertine Compulsion, it also has absolutely no impact upon the likelihood that they will kill. To understand the former, we need to understand that the moral emotions are products of evolution by natural selection. And, left undisturbed, will cause a person to act morally even if they do not deliberate on their actions—I do not kidnap, whether I think about it or not. However, a person with a

Libertine Compulsion acts immorally compulsively and cannot contain their urge because it is constant and never abates. To change this, we need to work on finding therapies that specifically target the nature of the emotions that have become corrupted.

'Responsibility' is a myth that is a corollary to the myth of free will. If I do something idiotic and then say 'I take responsibility for what I did', then this is an *ex post facto* recognition of the fact that I just did something in the recent past—a tautological explanation that says nothing about why I did it. If *you* do something idiotic, and I say 'I hold you responsible', then I am merely asserting my right to punish you. Again—nothing is explained as to why you did it. Our urge to punish comes not from reason, but from our biological make-up: anger is a biological mechanism for punishing people who do not fulfil their social obligations, and we can see this functioning in the chimpanzee society—an effective biological mechanism for making sure that everybody does what they are supposed to do. However, this does not work in a libertine compulsive because the operation of their biological mechanisms is corrupt. This is not just a deduction from this theory; it appears to be supported by the evidence. Extensive studies demonstrate that the death penalty does not reduce rates of homicide.[169] And jurisdictions with harsh criminal penalties do not have lower rates of criminality. There is even some statistical support for the view that the relationship is the other way round.

The urgency of tackling these problems is that the benefits are so extraordinarily wide. We reduce self-destructiveness and destructiveness at the same time. We do not like to admit it, but we mainly apply economic considerations in deciding strategies for managing the mad: medicine, talk therapy or prison. Rich people are given talk therapy because they have the money to pay for it and are easily exploited by the psychiatric profession. Poor people are given pills because it is cheaper than talk therapy. But ultimately, significant numbers of poor people who are given short shrift by the medical profession because of their inability to pay end up in prison. Sadly, this is the most expensive way of managing them. Because medical insurers or the government will not pay for talk therapy, the government ends up paying for prison instead. The short-sightedness of politicians has meant that, for society as a whole, we have adopted both the most expensive and the most inhumane solution.

Much of my work is seeking to show that a human action is the output of a calculation. Self-destructive actions are rational and madness is merely self-destruction squared. The actions of the mad are also the output of a calculation. Mental illness and criminality need to be seen as closely interrelated problems. This has a consequence that is difficult to accept: we need to show equal compassion to those that harm themselves and those that harm others because both are the result of similar mechanisms. Incarceration should be seen, not as punishment—since it has almost no deterrent value as such, but as a means of protecting society from people who are compelled to do harm. The primary goal of incarceration should be rehabilitation, and the type of institution in which we place people—jail or hospital—should be based upon which best fulfils this primary purpose. People who perform violent or antisocial actions because of a Libertine Compulsion or a Proactive Impulsion, should not be jailed for fixed periods based on the amount of harm they have caused in the past; they should be sent to treatment facilities for indeterminate periods. How long they are held should be based upon their therapists' judgement of whether their condition has improved rather than a legal judgement of how long is considered appropriate punishment for their actions. This approach is not without its own risks. In particular, therapists are likely to be reluctant to release mentally ill offenders even when their condition has improved for fear of being blamed for any subsequent reoffence.

Now that I have made the slightly provocative statement that 'responsibility' is a myth, I now need to address this question in more detail. It has been a long journey, but we are now equipped to look more generally at the causality of a human action and the moral questions that this throws up.

THE CALCULATION OF A HUMAN ACTION

Harris and Dennett view religion like a mental illness—imaginary friends, delusional beliefs, repetitive rituals, etc. Since I find this comparison to be particularly unhelpful, let me throw it straight back at them: if someone washes their hands for hours despite there being no need to do so and there being no improvement in cleanliness, we call it 'obsessive-compulsive disorder'; but if we ask the same question for two thousand years without it having any scientific relevance and without any progress in understanding or convergence upon consensus, we call it 'philosophy'. Dennett believes that the concept of free will is useful, but he cannot tell us what it is, and Harris argues that human actions are determined, but he cannot tell us how.

I hope that I am now in a position to state how a human action is determined or 'calculated' as I prefer to say. An emotion is a biological mechanism that causes an action state. But a human is the only animal on planet earth that has the intellectual capacity to out-think this mechanism. Does this make us 'free' while a chimpanzee is a prisoner of his pre-coded reaction to every situation?

An emotion turns a stimulus into a conscious urge to perform an action that we could hypothetically say has a 'value'. Critically, the reason that this is a philosophical problem, rather than a scientific one, is that scientists cannot measure the value of any emotion—that is only known to the person who has it. However, an advanced vertebrate will compare all the values of the different emotions that it feels at any moment and this results in an action based upon which urge is the strongest. It is worth tabulating the emotions to remind us how many such functions there are (Table 8). Taking this book and *The Logic of Self-Destruction*, I have mentioned most of them at some point:

TABLE 8: A SUMMARY OF HUMAN EMOTIONS

Emotion group or type	Driving emotion	Inhibiting emotion
Basic survival	Revulsion: recoil from noxious substances Pain: recoil from causes of bodily damage Fear: run away from imminent threat Hunger: seek adequate nutrition Thirst: remain hydrated	Tiredness: rest when energy levels are depleted Cannibalism taboo: do not eat your relatives Freeze: if you see a predator first
Reproduction	Humiliation: attack threats to biological fitness Jealousy: shield partner from rivals Lust: mate with fertile partner Nurture: Love of offspring Brotherly love: even your nieces and cousins carry some of your genes	Incest taboo: do not mate with close relatives
Social emotions	Pity: assist those in need, and keep a mental note of those that reciprocate Sympathy: consider how to avoid the difficulties faced by others Guilt: perform onerous social obligations Gratitude: bond with those that assist Loneliness: seek pack or herd and stay with them Anger: punish those who cheat in the performance of social obligations	Shame: do not perform asocial actions, even for your benefit
Strategic emotions	Anxiety: plan avoidance of hypothetical threats Sadness: consider what is not working and change it	Regret: do not repeat failed strategies

Plenty of people will quibble with my list. For example, I have left out grief because I cannot see that it has a biological function. Grief may be a subset of sadness—a failed strategy that ended with the death of someone important to you. I intentionally left out happiness because, like grief, it is not possible to think of an evolutionary origin or a biological function. I consider it to be an invented emotion.[170] I have also left out romantic love because I think it is a belief rather than an emotion. There are some pretty weird things that we could consider including on this list, such as, the urge to urinate, the urge to scratch, or the compulsion to worry with your tongue a bit of food stuck between your teeth—three emotional drivers that do not even have English names.

From the list of emotions in Table 8, all of these emotions are present in chimpanzees with the probable exception of the strategic emotions. Most of the social emotions are widespread in advanced social mammals, but presumably not in solitary animals. Most social mammals below the level of primate almost certainly lack the incest taboo. This is partly because the concept of 'sibling' requires an understanding of triadic relationships: 'that is my mother, and this is another creature that has the same mother'. We can demonstrate that primates understand triadic relationships, but it is probable that lower mammals cannot. With no understanding of the concept of sibling, red deer, lions and elephants eliminate the risk of inbreeding by the single expedient of expelling male members of the pack or herd as soon as they reach sexual maturity. Male primates generally stay within their troupe when mature.

Darwin explained the evolutionary origin of the basic survival and reproductive emotions, but he could not work out the evolutionary origin of all the others. W. D. Hamilton laid the foundations for our understanding of the mechanism for the evolution of the social emotions in 1964. This is so recent, that the implications of this are only just starting to trickle into philosophy. It is easy to imagine that science happens fast, but the transfer of ideas back and forth between science and philosophy is slow. Philosophers generally talk of the 'moral emotions' which is my list of social emotions but excluding anger and, possibly, loneliness. I believe that anger belongs in this list, since there is little point of separating driving our own pro-social actions from our reaction to the failure of others to perform theirs. All the social emotions act together to create a stable equilibrium among social vertebrates where everybody performs their social duties and nobody performs antisocial actions. This is clear when we observe chimpanzees, but less so when we observe humans. I suggest that the reason for this is that humans perform tactical deceptions with their emotional behaviour and the whole biological mechanism becomes confused by our out-thinking of our own biology.

Not long ago, we thought that neuroscience would provide answers to very old philosophical questions about free will and mind, but actually it did no such thing. Instead, neuroscientists all thought that they had to become philosophers, which generally made these problems even more annoying. In my opinion, it is the field of animal cognition that throws most light on how humans calculate actions. In the early 1980s, it was not in vogue for a biologist to suggest that animals *understood* things. If we ignore what chimpanzees understand, it makes it easier for us to blithely assume that we have free will and they do not. Now, the pendulum has swung too far the other way and sometimes biologists ascribe comprehension to animals that should provoke philosophical doubt. Despite this, recent research makes it pretty clear that the computation of an action in an advanced primate like a chimpanzee can be surprisingly complex. Consider this observation of de Waal in chimpanzees:

We had hidden some grapefruit in the chimpanzee enclosure. ... The chimpanzees knew what we were doing, because they had seen us go outside carrying a box full of fruit and they had seen us return with an empty box. The moment they saw that the box was empty they began hooting excitedly. As soon as they were allowed outside they began searching madly but without success. A number of apes passed the place where the grapefruits were hidden without

noticing anything—at least, that is what we thought. Dandy too
had passed over the hiding place without stopping or slowing
down at all and without showing any undue interest. That after-
noon, however, when all the apes were lying dozing in the sun,
Dandy stood up and made a bee-line for the spot. Without hesita-
tion he dug up the grapefruits and devoured them at his leisure. If
Dandy had not kept the location of the place a secret, he would
probably have lost the grapefruits to the others.[171]

There is a lot going on in this simple event. Firstly, Dandy suppresses
whatever reaction he might have had upon seeing the hidden grapefruit. Despite the aforementioned need for philosophical doubt, I
think it pretty clear that Dandy was deploying tactical deception. It is
worth breaking down what this requires: (1) he has a concept of his
own behaviour; (2) he understands that others react to his behaviour
in certain predicable ways; (3) if he changes his behaviour, others will
react to him differently; and (4) he can do this modification to make
the others reaction advantageous to him. There are at least four com-
ponents to this calculation, and a chimpanzee has the cognitive
capability to perform this. Dandy is suppressing behaviour (not
reacting when he sees the grapefruit) and this is a less complex deception than affecting behaviour. The latter is probably beyond a
chimpanzee's capability. He is also, strictly speaking, not performing
tactical deception with his emotional behaviour—something that
only humans can do fluently. Dandy also appears to demonstrate a
chimpanzee's capacity to conceive of the near-term future, since he is
intentionally deferring gratification. Prior to 1980, few people would
have believed that a chimpanzee could do these things.

Clearly, Dandy is performing a complex calculation. But does
this mean that he has free will? He is putting together all of the following elements: hunger, pleasure, his own behaviour, the past
reaction of other chimpanzees when he alone possesses food, and
the expectation that soon all the other chimpanzees will be distracted or sleepy. And he calculates the course of action that has the
best possible outcome for his own interest. It is unreasonable to

follow a path other than the best one, so the question of choice seems meaningless. It is a calculation; not a choice.

Let us now apply this thinking to humans and consider how emotions determine actions in humans. Humans have common ancestors with chimpanzees and have all the same emotional drivers (maybe plus a couple of extras) and a whole heap of additional cognitive capability. Consider, for example, the distinction between sympathy, empathy and compassion. To me, these have different meanings. I regard sympathy is the recognition of another's suffering or weakness as a result of one's own experience of these things. Empathy is the ability to recognise in another suffering or weakness that one has not experienced through projection onto the circumstances of the other. And compassion is the recognition of weakness or suffering in another despite no comparable experience. For example, a recovering alcoholic can sympathise the cravings of an alcoholic, but someone who is not an alcoholic can only empathise—if they have had a comparable experience—or show compassion if they have not. Compassion is the realm of the strong, since the weak can sympathise with everything. It is doubtful that a chimpanzee can recognise such nuance, principally because they lack language to describe their experiences. I cannot see that this additional nuance means that humans gain free will as a result. It simply means that a human is performing a more subtle calculation. For free will to suddenly spring into existence, we need to consider the changes from a chimpanzee to a human that are step-changes, rather than additional layers of nuance. The following are capabilities that humans have which chimpanzees probably lack:

- Language.
- Understanding of future emotions.
- Tactical deception with emotional behaviour, particularly affectation.
- Thinking about thinking.
- Morality.

Some might disagree that chimpanzees cannot do these things, but I am not sure that makes much difference to my argument since that would just push the dividing line where free will comes into being lower down the evolutionary tree. Let us consider whether any of these stops a human action being a result of a calculation. If it does, then maybe we can consider what 'free will' might mean. The difficulty is that all of these capabilities are interrelated and most are only possible because of language. But I do not think any philosopher thinks that free will is a function of language. It gives us the ability to think more complex thoughts and understand more abstract concepts. Chimpanzees have a limited capacity to understand the future and their own emotions, but probably not at the same time. The example of Dandy and the grapefruit makes it clear that a chimpanzee can suppress behaviour and de Waal also describes a situation where a chimpanzee suppressed emotional behaviour by manipulating his face with his fingers.[172] But I can find no evidence that a chimpanzee can affect emotional behaviour. It is difficult to overstate the impact of an ability to form concepts of future emotion, since it is the foundation upon which human reason is based. This is how Rousseau expressed it in the eighteenth century:

> It is by the activity of the passions that our reason is improved; for we desire knowledge only because we wish to enjoy; and it is impossible to conceive any reason why a person who has neither fears nor desires should give himself the trouble of reasoning. The passions, again, originate in our wants, and their progress depends on that of our knowledge; for we cannot desire or fear anything, except for the idea we have of it, or from the simple impulse of nature.[173]

I would go further in saying that ideas of *future* emotion are a prerequisite of reason. If one of our ancestors realised that tomorrow the sabre-toothed tiger might come to the cave, then that is not sufficient reason to do anything about it. However, this is a sufficient reason: the realisation that tomorrow the sabre-toothed tiger might come to the cave *and he will be frightened of it*. This is a prerequisite of building a barricade over the cave—perhaps the first application of reason by early hominids. The development of agriculture is often cited as the earliest step in human civilisation. But this required an understanding that food was plentiful in summer and scarce in winter. Agriculture would never have been developed without an understanding of future hunger at least six months in advance—almost certainly beyond the future horizon for a chimpanzee, and therefore a critical realisation for an early hominid. You go to the supermarket in advance of needing to eat because you have an understanding of future hunger. And this has a striking impact on the causality of a human action. In a chimpanzee, the emotion pushes the action, but a human is calculating an action to bring about future emotional outcomes. But Dandy is pushing against this boundary. The extent of his understanding is that if he digs up the grapefruit now, they will be taken off him anyway, so he might as well wait a bit to see if he can eat them later. He cannot alter the reaction of other chimpanzees by affecting behaviour and he is only looking into the very near-term future. But do the relatively advanced capabilities of a human stop their actions being the result of a calculation? The first human who realised that by gathering more food than he needed in summer, he could avoid hunger in winter was performing a very calculated action. And the suggestion that this was a choice is ludicrous because once you have worked it out it is absurd not to do it. If you do not do it because you are lazy, then that just means that your wish to slouch around has a higher value to you than your anxiety about future hunger. Still a calculation!

The ability of humans to perform tactical deception with their emotional behaviour means that they derive false understandings of their own emotions. When they work out what action to perform now to achieve a future emotional goal, they will deduce a self-destructive action. This is something that a chimpanzee could not manage, but it is still a calculation. It is a rational derivation of an action that ends up being self-destructive because it was derived from false information. So when humans do crazy stuff, it is not evidence that their actions are not rationally calculated.

Proponents of free will usually claim that children and the mad do not have it (whatever 'it' is). For example, Dennett recently claimed that: 'Infants don't have free will; normal adults do'.[174] However, in saying this, he is placing upon himself a heavy burden of proof of stating when free will springs into life (Weaning from the breast? Puberty? Twenty-first birthday?). He also needs to describe the process of it coming into being. An adult chimpanzee has a higher capacity to think than an infant child, but this is just a calculation of its best strategy in every situation. I hope that, in this book, I have destroyed the idea that the sane have free will and mad people do not; not by trying to prove that mad people do indeed have free will, but rather that they calculate their actions using the same mechanisms that the rest of us do. It is just that they are starting with a set of inputs that means that the output of the calculation repetitively ends up as a self-destructive action.

Let us consider thinking about thinking. Most animal cognition experts think that this is something that animals cannot do, but there are some dissenters. Self-doubt is the most obvious example of a human thinking about thinking. Even if a chimpanzee is capable of this (which I doubt), then the human still has a trump card because I can think about *you* thinking. Dandy can pretend not to see the hidden grapefruit because he knows what the other chimpanzees will *do* if he reveals their location. He does not need to know what they *think*. But the ability to do this raises the level of complexity immensely. Two grandmasters playing chess are each thinking out to several iterations 'if I do this, then he will probably think that by doing that he will force me to do the other . . .' But nobody doubts that they are calculating. Once they have worked out what they think is the best move (even when they make a mistake), then performing any other is absurd, so it is also absurd to suggest that that move is a choice. The loser is the one who fails to see what the other might do, or who cannot think as many moves into the future. This is a calculation limited by the ability to visualise and only run a finite number of iterations in your head. Calculating an action involves also performing a hypothetical calculation of the action of another, and this takes the process into the territory of game theory: two strategies face off against one another—still a calculation, but one where most of us are struggling because our ability to visualise surpasses our ability to compute. John Nash received a Nobel Prize for demonstrating that every game theoretical situation has a single calculable optimal strategy.[175] I can visualise some of the things that you might do that limit my strategy, but I cannot accurately compute which action you will perform because I am not aware of all your inputs. The calculation necessarily becomes one that involves estimates, probabilities and guesses. Still a calculation!

Humans perform tactical deception and presume that others do too. A chimpanzee can perform a tactical deception in a limited way, but probably cannot presume that another chimpanzee is doing this as an input to its own calculation. Two humans, by contrast, can be involved in a negotiation where both are lying and both presume that the other is lying. I once had a boss who was a compulsive liar. And I rather enjoyed it. I learned to spot his tells and dealing with him became a game because I did not suffer personally from his deceit: I was paid to be his pawn.

Our ability to out-think our own emotions, perform tactical deceptions and think about thinking makes this process iterative. But every computer scientist knows that iterative processes have determined outcomes. If an iterative process to calculate something never ends, then the person in whose head that process occurs cannot truly be said to be in control of that process since it never reaches a conclusion. If it does end, then the process produces an answer, and if the person questions that answer they are merely putting another iteration onto the end of the process. Ending the process of iteration is not a choice. At some point we have to do something and that creates a pressure to end the process of deciding what to do. The number of iterations we can perform is itself calculated. I spent five years over the decision to leave finance and become a writer. (With hindsight, I wish I had decided sooner.) I spend five seconds over the decision to have another beer. (Sometimes, with hindsight, I wish I spent longer.) Circumstances dictate different degrees of urgency (immediate threat or not), different degrees of momentousness (divorce will change the rest of your life, deciding whether to floss or just brush your teeth will not), and different degrees of complexity (significant investment decisions versus choosing the colour of your shirt each morning). You perform an iterative calculation where these circumstances dictate how many iterations of the calculation you can afford to perform. In other words, you calculate the number of iterations. This is no different to an iterative computer programme where the degree of the accuracy of the answer (and hence the number of iterations) is itself separately determined.

So, I have explained that a human action is the result of a calculation involving probability theory, guesses and estimates, iterative processes, game theory, deductions from false data and much more. But does this really happen? What if you are rubbish at mathematics? How do you survive in the human jungle? Worry Not! Nature has provided you with a computational substitute. In fact it is the same computational substitute used by a chimpanzee that cannot do mathematics at all. It's called an emotion. It returns a value for a given set of circumstances and simplifies the calculation for the mathematically challenged. For example, when you decide to marry someone—perhaps your most momentous decision—you can shortcut most of the mathematics. Trust is a value calculated from the cumulative memory of who has treated you well—not just history, but clues as to the type of people who can be predicted to do this. Suspicion is a value calculated from the cumulative memory of situations where you have been betrayed. A decision to marry is based on a blended average of these values plus lust, fear of loneliness and a quick assessment of their bank balance and personal hygiene. This is still a calculation—part intellectual and part reading the output of nature's computing device: the emotion. The illusion of choice is that you can read the answer and second-guess it. But deciding to stop doing this is also a calculation. If you do not stop it, life will pass you by and all your options will evaporate. Delay deciding beyond a critical point and fate decides for you.

Let us apply this situation to someone with a mental disorder. An alcoholic calculates their next action and the answer comes back that they should have a drink. They then second-guess the answer. 'No that cannot be the right answer!' so they perform the calculation again; and still the answer comes back that they should have a drink. This will keep repeating until eventually they have the drink. Someone who is a serial killer spends weeks or months performing a similar calculation, rejecting the answer and then getting the same answer again.

We now have one last human capability to consider: morality. This one causes particular philosopher angst because if we toss free will in the trash can, then the concept of responsibility goes with it. But few philosophers have fully absorbed that the moral emotions are part of our hardwiring.[176] Compassion has recently been demonstrated in laboratory rats[177] and is frequently anecdotally noted in dogs, monkeys and lions. You can find videos on the internet of a tortoise rolling another that is stuck on its back, so it is possible that compassion even exists in reptiles. So what is this 'morality' that humans are so proud of? Like any other emotion, you can out-think a moral emotion. A beggar can act pitiable (a tactical deception) to provoke your emotion of pity. And if you suspect that he or she is doing this intentionally, you might suppress the emotion of pity in return (also a tactical deception). Chimpanzees possess all the moral emotions that humans do, but they lack the ability to perform tactical deception with them and therefore do not need to think about them. A chimpanzee sees another member of its troupe in difficulty and helps without second-guessing its reaction. Humans have the urge to respond and understand the point of the urge. A morality is a belief about when you should apply or dis-apply a moral emotion. But in *Part II: Irrefutable Thoughts* of *The Logic of Self-Destruction* I demonstrated that beliefs are logical traps from which we cannot escape—hardly a choice then![178] The idea that we choose our beliefs is incoherent, since we believe them because we think they are *right*.

Furthermore, I demonstrated that all beliefs ultimately become destructive to the people who believe them. And this applies to moralities too.

Religious leaders claim that without religious teaching we would have no morality. What a fantastic outcome that would be! Secular societies are more peaceable and have lower rates of crime. If you doubt this, check the Global Peace Index where the top is dominated by predominantly secular societies from the Nordic region plus Austria, New Zealand, Switzerland, Canada and Japan. The bottom six nations (Sudan, Somalia, Iraq, South Sudan, Afghanistan and Syria,) are almost exclusively Muslim.[179] Christian nations populate the middle ground. Another measure that uses a different methodology but generates very similar results is the World Civility Report.[180] The surprising exception here is that Costa Rica leaps to the top of the table (presumably because it has no armed forces). Currently, the Islamic State is aspiring to enforce the ultimate morality: the purest form of Islam. But somehow, it all turned to genocide. It really would be better for all concerned if they did not bother! But what they are doing is not a choice either. Explaining the logic of belief systems that have the characteristics of mental illnesses will be the subject of the future final part of *The Logic of Self-Destruction* series.

If you have moral emotions, then you do not need a morality. You just need the wisdom to know when another is playing tactical deception with his own moral emotional behaviour. If the emotion of pity drives you to help an old lady to cross the road and the emotion of shame stops you stealing her handbag, then this does not make you a 'good' person; merely a normal one. Your action is a calculation based on the value returned by each of your emotions, including your moral ones. And just because someone else acts differently, it does not make it a choice.

THE PSYCHIATRY OF THE FUTURE

People hate it when you point out problems without coming up with solutions. They accuse you of 'negativity'. But this thinking often preserves delusions that everything is OK, when it is not. This book has sought to define a problem, but not give a solution. Doctors like to call this problem 'mental illness', but I just call it madness. I do not think it is an illness, and saying it is 'mental' does not clarify what it is either. I am trying to demonstrate that, even if someone has nothing wrong with their body or brain on a physico-chemical level, they can still be mad. But does this change anything for a psychiatrist? He or she still has to go to the office every day, where there will be a caseload of deeply self-destructive humans, where most have something wrong with them and where fixing them is still difficult. Some of them are manageable, but most are probably incurable in the sense that they will never be able to lead contented productive lives without intervention by doctors and social workers and continuing support from their families.

The history of psychiatry consists of long periods of despondency, interrupted by brief periods of hope. The periods of hope stemmed from ideas that redefined what it was to be human. The Renaissance was a reorientation of our world view as centred on humanity, rather than the divine. And this was the beginning of the end of the idea that madness was an affliction sent by God. During the Age of Enlightenment, it appeared that everything could be observed empirically and analysed rationally. This was the beginning of the scientific approach to understanding madness. By studying the mad, we could define what their problem was and could come up with a scientific description—or so it seemed. Romanticism was the inspiration for the natural emergence of the earliest days of psychiatry as a medical discipline. Nature was a cure from the anti-nature that was a product of man and his society. The asylum was to be a place of retreat, with clean air and where the mad could wander freely to relieve themselves of the burden that society had placed upon them. Such views were widely accepted in the early nineteenth century. Then Freud taught us that we should stop thinking of the mad as a sort of 'other', but should accept the madness that was in us all. The way that madness was discussed changed: it was divorced from its supposed foundations in sin.

Most recently, psychopharmacology told us that we could fix the problem with chemistry and technology. And since we had just sent a man to the moon, we were bursting with confidence that we could conquer anything and that the boffins would soon work it all out. This confidence has slowly faded into a realisation that we can take the most disturbed people, and make their most alarming behaviours disappear with chemistry without necessarily solving their disturbance. This has led to a cynicism within both psychiatry and the government. The government is looking for the cheapest way to tame its most troublesome citizens, and psychiatrists are frequently confronted with a conflict of interest: they take the government's money to make unmanageable people malleable to conform to a government objective while really knowing that there is little that they can do to help the patient. Many therapists will willingly treat a troubled patient for years while intentionally cultivating a relationship of dependency. From the beginning of the age of psychopharmacology, governments throughout the developed world have sought to close expensive mental hospitals and replace them with cheap community care. They then slowly strangle the community care in sequential budget cuts. People with severe mental health problems do not tend to vote, so they are easily disenfranchised in a democratic society. Inevitably, politicians want community care to consist of brief, inexpensive meetings with professionals that hand out prescriptions. Very disturbed people are then left to roam unsupervised until an almost inevitable interaction with the police sees them end in prison. This costs the same as a mental hospital, but without any of the necessary support. In America today, the percentage of the total population that is mentally ill and in prison is approximately the same as that of mental hospital inpatients in the 1950s. However, we should not be totally cynical about psychiatry's lack of progress. Many psychiatrists think that acute personality disorder is untreatable, but dialectical behaviour therapy has some success in treating borderline personality disorder. It does this by deconstructing the patient's understanding of his or her emotions and rebuilding this understanding one piece at a time. This is precisely the approach that I would predict would work, but it is extremely expensive, labour-intensive and time-consuming. Part of the reason for this is that the therapist likely cannot determine which emotion is the subject of the misconception. If we could pinpoint that, we could save a lot of time and effort by narrowing the focus of therapy to precisely the problem and nothing else.

The Logic of Self-Destruction series is seeking to redefine what it is to be human. We can reduce all the human sciences to logic and evolutionary theory. A human is a logical computational device that goal-seeks emotional outcomes. Self-destructive actions are not irrational. They are derived rationally because the mechanism self-references when a human impersonates his or her own behaviour. This quirk arises because humans are the only animals on this planet that have the intellectual capacity to out-think their own biology. And, as such, they are capable of forming circular causality with some very weird and self-destructive outcomes. Madness is the logical outcome of this process, or of deductions made from ideas of emotion that are misconceptions of a compound nature—involving more than one emotion at the same time. This is like a computer programme with a loop in it caused by the programme self-referencing.

Assuming that my analysis starts to gain traction in psychiatric and scientific circles, I expect a sequence of consequences. Firstly, researchers in the field of mental illness will start to interpret their findings in the light of this theoretical approach. I would hope that, if this type of interpretation leads to explanations of what we can observe falling neatly into place, then this will lead to a gradual consensus that this book does indeed describe the causal structure of many forms of madness, perhaps most of them. Secondly, we can start to derive better diagnostic tools. I would expect these to be worked out mathematically and they would enable us to specify exactly which emotion was being misunderstood, or which emotional behaviour was being manipulated. This should lead to the development of new therapies. I would predict that these would be talk therapies that would focus much more narrowly than has been possible in the past. Rather than having to build the entire history of the patient, we could identify quickly what is being misunderstood and what needs to be relearned. I believe that these therapies will be talk therapies that will be based in the mechanics of emotional functioning. The stock question of the psychotherapist 'how did that make you feel?' will disappear, since feelings are irrelevant to how a person functions. Instead, we will seek to rebuild people's understanding of their emotions by describing observable causes and effects of human responses to their environment. This will involve re-teaching the names of those emotions that are being misidentified, rehearsing the appropriate emotional behaviour based upon their Biological Stimuli, identifying the appropriate causes of emotions that are being affected, and demonstrating the occurrence of the emotions that are being suppressed. Where an emotional behaviour has disappeared because it has become suppressed, we will have to teach it; and, initially, this will involve affecting it in the appropriate circumstances. This affectation will be repeated until it is habitual and then the appropriate behaviour for a given stimuli will become learned correctly for the right stimulus.

Talk therapy for people with acute psychiatric conditions is a painstaking process not dissimilar to teaching illiterate adults how to read. We are teaching old dogs new tricks, long after the ability to learn these things effortlessly has ossified. But if we can narrow down what we need to teach to a targeted misconception, this process can be greatly speeded up. Rather than reconstructing an entire broken human, we just have to reconstruct a single broken emotion or maybe a pair of them.

An inevitable consequence of this will be a steady drift away from chemical 'cures'. This is going to be a painful transition because the pharmacology industry has vast investments in chemical therapies and a huge lobbying infrastructure within government. Talking cures are expensive and somebody needs to pay for them. Mental illness causes poverty, so private care is never going to be adequate. The right approach needs the government to understand that madness costs them tens of billions of dollars a year in hospital treatment, lost productivity, incarceration, physical damage, increased levels of policing, etc. They need the confidence that investing in committed targeted talk therapy can convert a person who is a burden to society to someone who is able to provide for themselves, work, pay taxes, etc. This is a rare case of a consensus between a moral *and* an economic argument. It will take a long time to build this confidence, particularly since many governments are increasingly rejecting scientific advice on matters such as evolution, climate change and narcotics policy. It does not help that psychiatry has a rather long history of false promises and dramatic failures. The continuing failure of psychiatry as a project is in danger of leading to a return to beliefs rejected centuries ago: that mad people are moral degenerates who belong in prison, and who should never be released until they 'snap out of it' and repent.

Despite these difficulties, I am optimistic that a new understanding of madness can lead to a development of new therapies that enable people to permanently escape compulsive self-destruction. And we can look forward to a new age of hope that is sustainable.

A NEW KIND OF FREEDOM

In this book, I have demonstrated that 'free will' is a fiction, and a madman—who is a prisoner of himself—is actually thinking the same way as the rest of us. Does this mean that we are not free? Freedom can mean many things, and what often happens is that we use the word in different ways depending upon the circumstances. Most of us apply the term inconsistently without noticing our contradictions. For example, some people think you should be free to let your children die by choosing not to vaccinate them, but you should not be free to choose an abortion. This raises the question about what freedom is, when you should have it and when it should be restricted. Currently, I am writing in the Lao People's Democratic Republic—a country that most westerners would presume is not free. However, Laos barely bothers to have laws and is so free that I sometimes wish that they would clamp it down a bit. For example, we could use a law around here that ten-year-olds cannot ride motorbikes without helmets. You might think me an orientalist, neo-colonial oppressor for suggesting such a thing, but Laos is a country with very high rates of road-traffic fatalities, and I think it is demonstrable that such a law would serve the greater good of the people, even though it confiscates a little piece of freedom. In most countries that regard themselves free, you are forbidden from riding a motorbike without a helmet (not just ten-year-olds). The justification for this is a concept of the greater good—a balance of the evil of loss of freedom and the probability of harming yourself. I think this the right policy. But it is fundamentally rooted in the recognition of the human capacity to self-destruct—effectively the government grants itself the right to protect you from yourself.

So, freedom does not in general mean that you can do what you want. It does not even mean that the government cannot tell you what you should not do. However, there are some things that we are very keen that the government cannot forbid us. In George Orwell's 1984, the government sought to forbid certain types of thoughts. But we recognise that no real government would seek to do such a thing because it is not practical. But there are plenty of real governments that tell you what you cannot say. Many governments, including democratic ones, forbid you to deny the Holocaust. In Thailand, you cannot criticise the King, and in Myanmar, you cannot criticise the military (which is almost the same thing as the government). Sometimes the implications of a prohibition are a bit difficult to pin down, so if the government of Iran declares you an 'enemy of God' that is pretty much the worst thing which they can accuse you of, but it really means that you are saying bad things about members of the government that have declared themselves the sole legitimate representatives of God. But then the Pope adopts this title too, but not (recently) in such an oppressive fashion. In countries like China and Turkey, there is a creeping prohibition on criticising the government. And in many countries, your ability to criticise the government may be officially permitted by freedom of speech laws, but there is an understanding that if you put it to the test, you might get a night-time visit from men in black balaclavas. America and Russia are both sliding down this path. If you are a white, middle-class person living in the West, you will no doubt smugly declare that your country is 'free' and you do not have any of these problems. But it is easy to think this, when you are an establishment figure who does not want to criticise the government because all governments do what is in the interest of establishment people. The delusion is that establishment people also generate the propaganda, so establishment people are free everywhere—assuming that they believe their own propaganda.

In countries that call themselves 'free', it is common for people to say that they are 'free to have their own opinion', but all too often this means that such people claim the right to not look at the evidence. People who are of the opinion that climate change is a hoax and evolution by natural selection is a lie are wilfully blind to the mountains of evidence that have been accumulated. This cuts both ways, people will only say that they 'respect your opinion', if they are confident that you are misinformed. I would never claim that I was free to have my own opinion because if I think something is true, I seek the appropriate evidence. Americans are free to hold the opinion that their country is free, but that opinion is almost certainly not supported by the facts.[181] Most Western democracies these days have laws against 'hate speech'. These are fine in theory, but generally not in practice because they are only applied when non-establishment people say bad things about establishment people and not the other way round. There comes to be an accepted way that establishment people can say bad things about non-establishment people, for example referring to them as radicals, terrorists, extremists or, in some cases, liberals or intellectuals. These distinctions and accepted terminologies are not written down, but are widely understood. In other words, Western governments that think of themselves as free implicitly tell you who you can hate and who you cannot. Clearly, if you state your hatred of establishment figures, then invisible barriers might start appearing in your life.

Maybe we should conclude that it is not practical or realistic to say that freedom means that you can do what you want, or that the government cannot tell you what you cannot do. So then, does freedom mean that the government cannot do certain things to you? Well, we now know that the government reads your emails and tracks your online activities. They might promise that they only read the emails of bad people, but we now have an accumulation of evidence that this promise is empty. The real danger is not that they can read the emails of people like you and me, but that some people in government can read the emails of anybody who regulates or controls them. They only need to destroy the reputation of a couple of such people (e.g. General Petraeus, the head of the CIA, or Eliott

Spitzer, a prominent prosecutor) to demonstrate that they have an ability to do so to anybody (e.g. Dianne Feinstein who chaired the committee responsible for regulating American government wire-tappers). When they exercise this power, it creates a fear where they become the establishment and nobody risks criticising them. This is how totalitarianism can exist in a nominally democratic society like Russia or Iran, and how America is slowly sliding towards such a state despite considering itself a beacon of freedom and democracy. Democracy is no guarantor of freedom.

Even the fundamentals of freedom, such as the writ of habeas corpus—the right not to be imprisoned without trial—are being eroded. Should we give up in despair then? The corrosion of Western liberalism is slowly progressing and we are all sliding down with it to an uncertain future that is almost sure to be less free than it is today.

I think we should not give up. I want you to consider a different form of freedom; one that is almost entirely within your control and, to my knowledge, is not written into the constitutional law of any nation, democratic or otherwise. I want you to consider freedom to mean that no one can tell you what you should *feel*.

Before, you can consider what this means, let us take a quick inventory of all the people who break this rule with no sense that they are doing wrong. Governments tell you that you should love your country because that makes you tame and easy to govern. They tell you that you should be stoic in the face of hard times and you should fear their enemies because otherwise you will blame them for the failure of their economic and foreign policies. My rule is that a government only tells you what you should feel when they do not know what to do in the face of an uncontrollable threat. Margaret Thatcher did not tell people what to feel because she always thought she knew what to do (even when she was wrong).

Priests tell you that true joy comes from worship and suffering will come to those that are not observant of their religion. The ludicrous fallacy of this is deduced from the clear incentive of the person who is doing the telling. Yoga teachers (who are high priests in mufti) constantly tell people what to feel. One once told me to 'send out love to all sentient beings'. OK, you're the teacher—demonstrate how that's done! Yoga classes these days often end with undisguised religious prayer sessions. The New Age warriors constantly talk about feelings while telling you that your feelings are whatever you want them to be. This is not freedom of expression, it is a dogma of meta-expression. They are walking away from formal religion and, by developing self-obsession to a heightened level, are creating a personal religion of themselves.

Waiters in New York City plonk your food on the table and order you: 'Enjoy!' It's none of their business whether I enjoy it or not. I might be deep in thought and not seeking any sensory experience from the food at all. However, they are just doing what everybody who is selling anything is doing—namely telling you how much emotional gratification you will obtain from their product. The advertising industry is telling you what to enjoy, not with words, but with behaviour: good looking actors pretend ecstasy while consuming the product being advertised; and ugly actors pretend to look stupid, confused or miserable while consuming any alternate product. This is a global conspiracy of lying. And it has an impact: cumulatively, it programmes you to define your well-being in terms of consumption. Humanity over-consumes. This is an ideology that will lead to the self-destruction of our species and most of the others with which we share our planet.

It takes discipline to ignore these signals. It is even harder if they crept into your childhood through manipulative adults. But once you recognise these patterns you can steer clear of them. Be candid about what you feel and forthright in your determination that nobody else can tell you what you ought to feel. When you feel pity, act on it! Do not pause to consider whether the subject of that pity is of your tribal group. When someone shows you altruism, do not consider how to manipulate your response of gratitude! When someone injures you, display your anger! Recognise that just because a human is a biological mechanism that does not mean that your feelings do not matter. It means that your feelings are the means by which you interact with other humans as the members of a social species. But globalisation and the media have now made that species a global tribe. A Palestinian is as much a member of your tribe as an Amazonian Indian. Recognition of this means that compassion—that ultimate urge to cooperate and coexist—spreads its tentacles across the global network that is humanity. And by treating all the rights of men equally, we can learn to live together without conflict and without the collective self-destruction of our species.

NOTES

1. Blakeway M. The Logic of Self-Destruction: The Algorithm of Human Rationality. York: Meyer LeBoeuf; 2014.
2. Harris S. The End of Faith: Religion, Terror and the Future of Reason. New York: WW. Norton; 2004.
3. Hunter R, Macalpine I. Three Hundred Years of Psychiatry: 1535–1860. A History Presented in Selected English Texts. London: Oxford University Press; 1963.
4. Foucault M. *History of Madness*. Trans. by Murphy J, Khalfa J. London and New York: Routledge; 2006, p. 473.
5. Ibid.
6. Ibid. pp. 190–1. Foucault cites Paracelsus, *Sämtlicke Werke*. Munich: Südhoff, 1923. '1 Abteilung, Vol. II', p. 391.
7. Burton R. *The Anatomy of Melancholy*. New York: New York Review of Books; 2001. 'The First Partition', p. 393.
8. Ibid. p. 273.
9. Ibid. p. 194.
10. Quoted in Lefkowitz MR, Fant MB. (eds.) *Women's Life in Greece and Rome: A Source Book in Translation*. 3rd ed. Baltimore: John Hopkins University Press; 2005, pp. 237–40.
11. Quoted in Porter R. Madness: *A Brief History*. Oxford: Oxford University Press; 2002, p. 46.
12. Castillo H. *Personality Disorder: Temperament or Trauma? An Account of an Emancipatory Research Study Carried Out by Service Users Diagnosed with Personality Disorder*. London and Philadelphia: Jessica Kingsley Publishers; 2003, p. 13.
13. Foucault M. op. cit., p. 193. Foucault gives the citation: K. Linné. *Genera Morborum*. Upsala; 1763.
14. Ibid. p. 278.
15. Hippocrates, *lib. de Insania et Melancholia*. Quoted in Burton R. op. cit., p. 387.

16. Szasz TS. *The Myth of Mental Illness: Foundations of a Theory of Personal Conduct*. Ebook. New York: Harper Collins; 1961. Kindle Location 874.

17. Plato. The Timeaus. In: Jowett M. (ed. and trans.) *The Dialogues of Plato, in Five Volumes, Vol III*. 3rd ed. London: Oxford University Press; 1892, p. 323.

18. Arkowitz H, Lilienfeld SO. Lunacy and the Full Moon: Does a Full Moon Really Trigger Strange Behavior? *Scientific American*. Website. 27 January 2009.

19. Burton R. op. cit., p. 213.

20. Ibid. p. 175.

21. Ibid. p. 173.

22. Ibid. pp. 300–30.

23. Ibid. p. 385.

24. Ibid. p. 419.

25. Foucault M. op. cit., pp. 183–4.

26. Hegel GWF. Philosophy of Mind. Trans.by Wallace W. *Blackmask Online*. 2001, § 408. Available from: http://www.hegel.net/en/pdf/Hegel-Enc3.pdf [Accessed 17 September 2015].

27. Foucault M. op. cit., p. 187. Foucault replicates the archaic spelling.

28. Ibid. p. 222

29. Ibid. p. 223. Foucault cites Esquirol, Vol. II, p. 219.

30. Ibid. pp. 282–3.

31. Porter R. *The Greatest Benefit to Mankind: A Medical History of Humanity from Antiquity to the Present*. London: Harper Collins; 1997, p. 508.

32. Guillain G. *J.-M. Charcot, 1825–1893, His Life—His Work*. Ed. and Trans. by Bailey P. London: Pitman Medical Publishing; 1959, p. 174. The author states that he visited Salpêtrière after Charcot's death and several of the patients perfectly imitated the symptoms of hysteria (note 11, p. 174). Also, an English physician, Axel Munthe, attended Charcot's lectures, which were more of a theatrical performance attended by society people. Munthe wrote that he suspected fraud on the part of Charcot's patients to ensure the desired theatrical effect during lectures (note 12, p. 174).

33. Popper KR. Conjectures and Refutations: The Growth of Scientific Knowledge. London: Routledge & Keagan Paul, 1963. Chapter 1, Science: Conjectures and Refutations, Section VII.

34. Eissler K. Malingering. In: Wilbur GB, Muensterberger W. (eds.) Psychoanalysis and Culture. New York: International Universities

Press; 1951, pp. 252–3. Quoted in Szasz TS. op. cit., Kindle Location 985.

35. Laing RD. *The Divided Self. An Existential Study in Sanity and Madness.* Intro. by David A. London: Penguin Books; 2010, p. 82.

36. Ibid. p. 141.

37. Foucault M. op. cit., pp. 297ff.

38. Ibid. pp. 305–6.

39. Torrey EF. *Out of the Shadows: Confronting America's Mental Illness Crisis.* New York: John Wiley & Sons; 1997.

40. Porter R. 1997, op. cit., p. 518.

41. Laing RD. op. cit., p. 160.

42. Higgins ES, George MS. *Neuroscience of Clinical Psychiatry: The Pathophysiology of Behaviour and Mental Illness.* 2nd ed. Philadelphia: Lippincott, Williams & Wilkins; 2013. Chapter 2: Neuroanatomy, p.18.

43. Von Wagner-Jauregg won in 1927 and Moniz won in 1949. Nobel Prize. List of all Nobel Laureates in Physiology or Medicine. *Nobelprize.org.* Nobel Media AB 2014. Website. Available from: http://www.nobelprize.org/nobel_prizes/medicine/laureates/ [Accessed 3 March 2015].

44. Quoted in Burton R. op. cit., p. 177.

45. Hirschfeld RMA, Vornik LA. Bipolar Disorder—Costs and Comorbidity. *The American Journal of Managed Care*, 2005; 11(suppl. 3), pp. S85–S90.

46. Szasz TS. op. cit. Kindle Location 393.

47. Szasz TS. op. cit. Kindle Location 3250. Opening paragraph of the Chapter 'Personality Development and Moral Values'.

48. Hare RD. *Without Conscience: The Disturbing World of the Psychopaths among Us.* New York: Guilford Press; 1999, p. 194.

49. Winerip M, Schwirtz M. Rikers: Where Mental Illness Meets Brutality in Jail. *The New York Times.* Website. 14 July 2014.

50. Schwirtz M. Rikers Island Struggles with a Surge in Violence and Mental Illness. *The New York Times.* Website. 18 March 2014.

51. A term used to reference people who get a prescription from their doctor that they intend to use as a narcotic as opposed to medical treatment.

52. Nisen M. The 10 Best Selling Prescription Drugs in the United States. *Business Insider.* Website. 28 June 2012. Available from: http://www.businessinsider.com/10-best-selling-blockbuster-drugs-2012-6?op=1 [Accessed 2 January 2014]

53. Foucault M. op. cit., p. 529 (Foucault's emphasis).

54. Ibid. p. 538.

55. Ryle G. *The Concept of Mind*. London: Penguin (Peregrine Books); 1978. Chapter X, Psychology, p. 296.

56. Wittgenstein L. *Lectures & Conversations on Aesthetics, Psychology and Religious Belief*. Oxford: Blackwell Publishing; 1966, p. 41.

57. Popper KR. op. cit., pp. 33–9.

58. A mathematician could describe a biological emotion as a function $f(C) = A$, where C is a set of circumstances and A is an action state. However, as Stephen Hawking once pointed out, every mathematical formula that you put in a book, halves its sales (quoted Gribbin J. The Thoughts of Stephen Hawking. *New Scientist*, No. 1621, 14 July 1988, p. 64).

59. Darwin C. *The Expression of Emotions in Man and Animals*. In: Wilson EO. (ed.) *From So Simple a Beginning: Darwin's Four Great Books*. New York: WW. Norton & Company; 2005.

60. Blakeway M. op. cit. The Engineering of Humiliation, pp. 278–303.

61. Blakeway M. op. cit. Part I: The Human Algorithm.

62. Blakeway M. op. cit. The Invention of Emotion, pp. 128–39.

63. Kierkegaard S. *Works of Love*. Trans. and eds. by Hong HV, Hong EH. Princeton, NJ: Princeton University Press; 1998, Volume 16.

64. Darwin C. On the Origin of the Species by Means of Natural Selection. In: Wilson EO. (ed.) *From So Simple a Beginning: Darwin's Four Great Books*. New York: WW. Norton & Company; 2005.

65. Darwin C. *The Descent of Man, and Selection in Relation to Sex*. op. cit.

66. Darwin C. *The Expression of Emotions in Man and Animals*. op. cit.

67. Hamilton WD. The Genetical Evolution of Social Behaviour. I. *Journal of Theoretical Biology*. 1964; 7(1), pp. 1–16.

68. de Waal F. *Chimpanzee Politics: Power and Sex among Apes*. Revised Edition 2000. Kindle Edition. Baltimore and London: John Hopkins University Press; 2007. Kindle Locations 246–249.

69. Ibid. Kindle Locations 1890–1894.

70. Ibid. Kindle Locations 2034–2038.

71. Confucius. *The Analects*. Trans. by Waley A. London, New York, Toronto: Everyman's Library; 2001, § 26.

72. Laing RD. op. cit. Preface to the second edition.

73. Blakeway M. op. cit. The Engineering of Humiliation. pp. 278–303.

74. Burton R. op. cit., 'The First Partition', p. 424.

75. W. D. Hamilton was the inventor of neither of the concepts of relatedness or the evolutionarily stable strategy, but he was most influential in exploiting them to develop new evolutionary theory.

76. Rothenbuhler WC. Behaviour Genetics of Nest Cleaning in Honey Bees. IV. Responses of F_1 and Backcross Generations to Disease-Killed

Brood. *American Zoologist.* 1964; 4(2): pp. 111–23. (I first learnt of this research from Dawkins R. *The Selfish Gene.* 30th anniversary ed. Oxford: Oxford University Press; 2006. Chapter 4, The Gene Machine.)

77. Dawkins R. *The Extended Phenotype.* Oxford: Oxford University Press; 1982.

78. Zhisui L. *The Private Life of Chairman Mao.* New York: Random House, Inc.; 1994.

79. According to the gene theory of Mendel, we can test a hypothesis that a single gene determines a characteristic by experimentally cross-breeding adults that do or do not have the characteristic and see which of their offspring have it. 'Breeding pure' means, depending on which parent has the gene on which chromosome, that the offspring will display the characteristic either 100 per cent, 0 per cent, 50/50 or 75/25 of the time.

80. Dawkins R. 1982, op. cit., the definition of 'altruism' is in the Glossary.

81. von Neumann J. The Mathematician. *Works of the Mind.* I(I). Chicago: University of Chicago Press; 1947, pp. 180–96.

82. Blakeway M. op. cit. for example, Scenario: The Moral Logic of Tyranny, pp. 183–5

83. Shephard B. *A War of Nerves; Soldiers and Psychiatrists, 1914–1994.* London: Jonathan Cape; 2000.

84. Sade Marquis de. *Justine, or the Misfortunes of Virtue.* Trans. by Phillips J. Oxford: Oxford University Press, Oxford World Classics; 2012. Introduction by Phillips J, p. xvi.

85. Hooker E. The Adjustment of the Male Overt Homosexual. *Journal of Projective Techniques.* 1957; 21, pp.18–31.

86. Gumert MD. Payment For Sex in a Macaque Mating Market. *Animal Behaviour.* 2007; 74(6), pp. 1655–67.

87. de Waal F. op. cit. Kindle Locations 308–310.

88. Kremer W. *The Evolutionary Puzzle of Homosexuality.* BBC World Service. Website. 18 February 2014.

89. Futuyma DJ, Risch SJ. Sexual Orientation, Sociobiology, and Evolution. *Journal of Homosexuality.* 1984; 9(2–3), pp. 157–68.

90. Blanchard R. Fraternal Birth Order and the Maternal Immune Hypothesis of Male Homosexuality. *Hormones and Behaviour.* 2001; 40(2), pp.105–14.

91. Rahman Q. The Association between the Fraternal Birth Order Effect in Male Homosexuality and Other Markers of Human Sexual Orientation. *Biology Letters.* 2005; 1(4), pp. 393–5.

92. Rahman Q, Hull MS. An Empirical Test of the Kin Selection Hypoth-

esis for Male Homosexuality. *Archives of Sexual Behavior.* 2005; 34(4), pp. 461–7.

93. de Waal F. op. cit. Kindle Location 1688.

94. The Kinsey Institute. *Frequently Asked Sexuality Questions to The Kinsey Institute.* Website. 2015. Available from: http://www.kinseyinstitute.org/resources/FAQ.html#Age [Accessed 4 November 2015].

95. Bailey JM. Book Review: Michael Jackson's Dangerous Liaisons. By Carl Toms. Padstow, Cornwall, TJ International, 2010. *Archives of Sexual Behavior;* 2011. DOI 10.1007/s10508-011-9842-1. Available from: http://faculty.wcas.northwestern.edu/JMichael-Bailey/articles/MJOCarrollReview.pdf [Accessed 25 October 2015]. See also: Sandfort T. *Boys on Their Contacts with Men: A Study of Sexually Expressed Friendships.* New York: Global Academic Publishers; 1987.

96. Best J. Age of Consent Should Be Lowered to 15, Argues Leading Health Expert. *Mirror Online.* Website. 17 November 2013. Available from: http://www.mirror.co.uk/news/uk-news/lower-age-consent-15-argues-2801227 [Accessed 17 March 2015].

97. Hooker E. op. cit.

98. Cantor JM, Kunban ME, Blak T, et al. Physical Height in Pedophilic and Hebephilic Sexual Offenders. *Sexual Abuse: A Journal of Research and Treatment.* 2007; 19(4), pp. 395–407.

99. Cantor JM, Klassen PE, Dickey R, et al. Handedness in Pedophilia and Hebephilia. *Archives of Sexual Behavior.* 2005; 34(4), pp. 447–59. See also: Blanchard R, Kolla NJ, Cantor JM, et al. IQ, Handedness, and Pedophilia in Adult Male Patients Stratified by Referral Source. Sexual Abuse: A Journal of Research and Treatment. 2007; 19(3), pp. 285–309.

100. Abel GG, Osborn C. The Paraphilias: The Extent and Nature of Sexually Deviant and Criminal Behavior. *Psychiatric Clinics of North America.* 1992; 15(3), pp. 675–87.

101. de Waal F. op. cit. Kindle Locations 1527–1530.

102. Wittgenstein L. *Philosophical Investigations.* Trans. by Anscombe GEM. Oxford: Basil Blackwell Ltd; 1953, §1. (Wittgenstein's reference: Augustine. *Confessions*, I.8.)

103. See, for example: Fonagy P, Luyten P. Psychodynamic Models of Personality Disorder. In: Widiger TA. (ed.) *The Oxford Handbook of Personality Disorders.* New York: Oxford University Press; 2012, pp. 345–371. Also: Bartholomew K, Kwong MJ, Hart SD. Attachment. In: Livesley WJ. (ed.) *Handbook of Personality Disorders: Theory, Research and Treatment.* New York and London: The Guilford Press; 2001, pp. 196–230.

104. Wittgenstein L. op. cit., 1953, §257.

105. Ibid. §288.

106. Ibid. §281.

107. Ibid. §ix. (Emphasis is Wittgenstein's.)

108. Ibid.

109. Blakeway M. op. cit. Part I: The Human Algorithm, p. 19.

110. Darwin C. *The Decent of Man*, op. cit. Chapter VIII, Principles of Sexual Selection.

111. Daly M, Wilson M. *Homicide*. New Brunswick, NJ: Transaction Publishers; 1988, pp.149–52.

112. de Fruyt F, de Clercqu B. Childhood Antecedents of Personality Disorders. In: Widiger TA. (ed.) *The Oxford Handbook of Personality Disorders*. New York: Oxford University Press; 2012, pp. 166–85.

113. Torgersen, S. Epidemiology. In: Widiger TA. (ed.) *The Oxford Handbook of Personality Disorders*. New York: Oxford University Press; 2012, pp. 186–205.

114. Laing RD. op. cit.

115. Fazel S, Danesh J. Serious Mental Disorder in 23,000 Prisoners: A Systematic Review of 62 Surveys. *The Lancet*. 2002, 359(9306), pp. 545–50. doi:10.1016/S0140-6736(02)07740-1 [Accessed 18 June 2015].

116. Torgersen S. op. cit.

117. Blashfield RK, Reynolds SM, Stennett B. The Death of Histrionic Personality Disorder. In: Widiger TA. (ed.) *The Oxford Handbook of Personality Disorders*. New York: Oxford University Press; 2012, pp. 603–27.

118. Harris S. 2004, op. cit.

119. Foucault M. op. cit., pp. 473ff.

120. Glynn I. *An Anatomy of Thought: The Origin and Machinery of the Mind*. Oxford: Oxford University Press; 1999, p. 347.

121. For example, Dennett describes a similar example of the evolution of endorphins and their receptors. Dennett DC. *Darwin's Dangerous Idea, Evolution and the Meanings of Life*. New York: Simon & Schuster; 1995, pp. 233ff.

122. Ball J. The Minnesota Starvation Experiment. *BBC World Service*. Website. 20 January 2014. Available from: http://www.bbc.co.uk/news/magazine-25782294 [Accessed 20 August 2015].

123. Levi P. *The Drowned and the Saved*. London: Abacus; 1989, p. 60.

124. Glynn I. op. cit., p. 346.

125. Ibid. p. 346.

126. Ibid.

127. Mitchell AJ, Selmes T. Why Don't Patients Take Their Medicine? Reasons and Solutions in Psychiatry. *Advances in Psychiatric Treatment.* 2007; 13(5), pp. 336–46.

128. Morrison AP, Turkington D, Pyle M. et al. Cognitive Therapy For People with Schizophrenia Spectrum Disorders Not Taking Antipsychotic Drugs: A Single-Blind Randomised Controlled Trial. *The Lancet.* 2014; 383(9926), pp. 1395–1403.

129. Scull A. A Convenient Place to Get Rid of Inconvenient People: The Victorian Lunatic Asylum. In: King AD. (ed.) *Buildings and Society: Essays on the Social Development of the Built Environment.* London, Routledge; 2005, pp. 19–31.

130. Foucault M. op. cit., p. 54.

131. Sade Marquis de. op. cit. Introduction, p. xiv.

132. Foucault M. op. cit., p. 50.

133. Ibid. p. 297.

134. Ibid. pp. 325–6.

135. Ibid. p. 325.

136. Ibid. p. 338.

137. Ibid. p. 359. Foucault quotes a priest called Desmonceaux from 1789.

138. Ibid. p. 400.

139. Ibid. p. 452.

140. Porter R. 2002, op. cit., p. 154.

141. Ibid. p. 155.

142. Foucault M. op. cit., p. 526.

143. Porter R. 1997, op. cit., p. 504.

144. Porter R. 2002, op. cit., p. 172.

145. Szasz TS. op. cit. Kindle location 177.

146. Castillo H. op. cit., p. 15.

147. Jokela M, Batty GD, Vahtera J, et al. Socioeconomic Inequalities in Common Mental Disorders and Psychotherapy Treatment in the UK between 1991 and 2009. *British Journal of Psychiatry.* 2013; 202(2), pp. 115–20.

148. Goldberg EM, Morrison SL. Schizophrenia and Social Class. *The British Journal of Psychiatry.* 1963; 109(463), pp. 785–802.

149. Saraceno B, Levav I, Kohn R. The Public Mental Health Significance of Research on Socio-Economic Factors in Schizophrenia and Major Depression. *World Psychiatry.* 2005; 4(3), pp. 181–85.

150. Torrey EF, Kennard AD, Eslinger DF, Biasotti BC, Fuller DA. *Justifiable Homicides by Law Enforcement Officers: What is the Role of Mental Illness?* Arlington, VA: Treatment Advocacy Center and the

National Sherrifs' Association; 2013. Available from: http://tacreports. org/storage/documents/2013-justifiable-homicides.pdf [Accessed 3 April 2015].

151. The Council of States Governments, Justice Center. *Improving Outcomes for People with Mental Illnesses Involved with New York City's Criminal Court and Correction Systems.* New York: Council of States Governments, Justice Center; 2012. Available from: http://csgjustice-center.org/wp-content/uploads/2013/05/CTBNYC-Court-Jail_7-cc. pdf [Accessed 26 November 2014].

152. The most up-to-date statistics that I can find on this are from 1999, which seems to imply that nobody seems to consider this matter worthy of updated academic research. Lymburner JA, Roesch R. The Insanity Defense: Five Years of Research (1993–1997). *International Journal of Law and Psychiatry.* 1999; 22(3–4), pp. 213–40.

153. Winerip M, Schwirtz M. op. cit.

154. Schwirtz M. op. cit.

155. Davis C. Under the Bridge: The Crime of Living without a Home in Los Angeles. *The Intercept.* Website. 25 July 2015. Available from: https://firstlook.org/theintercept/2015/07/25/criminalizing-homeless-ness-in-los-angeles/ [Accessed 28 July 2015]

156. Walmsley R. *World Pre-Trial/Remand Imprisonment List (Second Edition).* London: International Centre for Prison Studies; 2014. Available from: http://www.prisonstudies.org/sites/default/files/ resources/downloads/world_pre-trial_imprisonment_list_2nd_ edition_1.pdf [Accessed 16 June 2015].

157. Mosendz P, Reuters. Robert Durst's History of Skipping Bail Comes Back to Haunt Him. *Newsweek.* Website. 23 March 2015. Availablefrom:http://www.newsweek.com/robert-durst-jinx-denied-bail-316108 [Accessed 26 March 2015].

158. Torrey EF. op. cit.

159. Ibid.

160. For example: BBC News. US Gunman James Holmes 'Legally Sane' At Time of Shooting. *BBC News US & Canada.* Website. 29 May 2015. Available from: http://www.bbc.com/news/world-us-canada-32936495 [Accessed 30 May 2015 and 2 June 2015].

161. Porter R. 2002, op. cit., p. 155.

162. Ford M. America's Largest Mental Hospital Is a Jail. *The Atlantic.* Website. 8 June 2015. Available from: http://www.theatlantic.com/politics/ archive/2015/06/americas-largest-mental-hospital-is-a-jail/395012/ [Accessed 12 June 2015].

163. James DJ, Glaze LE. *Mental Health Problems of Prison and Jail Inmates. Bureau of Justice Statistics Special Report.* Washington, DC: U.S. Department of Justice; 2006. Available from: http://www.bjs.gov/content/pub/pdf/mhppji.pdf [Accessed 15 March 2015], p. 3.

164. United States Census Bureau. U.S. and World Population Clock. *United States Census Bureau.* Website. 2015. Available from: http://www.census.gov/popclock/ [Accessed 15 March 2015].

165. James DJ, Glaze LE. op. cit., p. 9.

166. Binelli M. Inside America's Toughest Federal Prison. *The New York Times Magazine.* Website. 26 March 2015. Available from: http://www.nytimes.com/2015/03/29/magazine/inside-americas-toughest-federal-prison.html?_r=0 [Accessed 28 March 2015].

167. Ibid.

168. Harris S. *Free Will.* Kindle Edition. New York: Free Press; 2012. Kindle location 573.

169. Lamperti J. *Does Capital Punishment Deter Murder? A Brief Look At the Evidence.* Hanover, NH: Dartmouth College; date unspecified. Available from: https://www.dartmouth.edu/~chance/teaching_aids/books_articles/JLpaper.pdf [Accessed 22 May 2015].

170. Blakeway M. op cit. The Invention of Emotion, pp. 128ff.

171. de Waal F. op. cit. Kindle Location 609.

172. de Waal F. op. cit. Kindle Location 1312.

173. Rousseau J-J. A Discourse on the Origin and Basis of Inequality amongst Men. In: Ryan A. (ed.), Cole GDH. (trans.) *The Social Contract and the Discourses.* London, New York, Toronto: Everyman's Library; 1993, pp. 31–126.

174. Dennett DC. Reflections on Free Will: A Review. *Sam Harris.* Weblog. 2014. Available from: http://www.samharris.org/blog/item/reflections-on-free-will [Accessed 27 January 2014], p. 13.

175. Nasar S. *A Beautiful Mind.* New York: Simon & Schuster; 1998

176. One of the most thorough surveys of evolutionary theory performed by a philosopher is in Dennett's *Darwin's Dangerous Idea: Evolution and the Meanings of Life*, which was published in 1995, barely 30 years after W. D. Hamilton explained the evolution of altruism. Not only (on my reading) does Dennett seem to miss the philosophical implications of moral emotions being products of evolution by natural selection, he does not say much about the meanings of life promised by his subtitle. (Dennett DC. 1995, op. cit.)

177. Ben-Ami Bartal I, Decety J, Mason P. Empathy and Pro-Social Behavior in Rats. *Science.* 2011; 334(6061), pp. 1427–30.

178. Blakeway M. op. cit. The Logic of Believing, pp. 151–72.
179. Arnett G. Global Peace Index 2014: Every Country Ranked. *The Guardian*. Website. 18 June 2014. Available from: http://www.theguardian.com/news/datablog/2014/jun/18/global-peace-index-2014-every-country-ranked [Accessed 12 March 2015].
180. Alavi M. *Civility Report 2014: Human Rights, Democracy, Peace, and Civility Analyses and Scores*. Katy, Texas: Peace Worldwide Organization; 2015. Available from: www.PeaceWorldwide.org [Accessed 12 March 2015].
181. For example, The World Civility Report, Alavi M. op. cit., ranks America in the third category 'harassment' out of nine in human rights (Table 4); and the third category out of ten for democracy (Table 6). On 'global peace', they are ranked in the same decile as North Korea and Afghanistan (Table 9).

BIBLIOGRAPHY

Abel GG, Osborn C. The Paraphilias: The Extent and Nature of Sexually Deviant and Criminal Behavior. *Psychiatric Clinics of North America*. 1992; 15(3): pp. 675–87.

Alavi M. *Civility Report 2014: Human Rights, Democracy, Peace, and Civility Analyses and Scores*. Katy, Texas: Peace Worldwide Organization; 2015. Available from: www.PeaceWorldwide.org [Accessed 12 March 2015].

American Psychiatric Association. *Diagnostic and Statistical Manual of Mental Disorders, Second Edition: DSM-II (Seventh Printing)*. Arlington, Virginia: American Psychiatric Publishing; 1974.

American Psychiatric Association. *Diagnostic and Statistical Manual of Mental Disorders, Third Edition: DSM-III*. Arlington, Virginia: American Psychiatric Publishing; 1980.

American Psychiatric Association. *Diagnostic and Statistical Manual of Mental Disorders, Fourth Edition: DSM-IV*. Arlington, Virginia: American Psychiatric Publishing; 1994.

American Psychiatric Association. *Diagnostic and Statistical Manual of Mental Disorders, Fifth Edition: DSM-V*. Arlington, Virginia: American Psychiatric Publishing; 2013.

Aristotle. *Nicomachean Ethics*: 2nd ed. Trans. by Irwin T. Indianapolis/Cambridge: Hackett Publishing Company, Inc.; 1999.

Arkowicz H, Lilienfeld SO. Lunacy and the Full Moon: Does a Full Moon Really Trigger Strange Behavior? *Scientific American*. Website. 27 January 2009. Available from: http://www.scientificamerican.com/article/lunacy-and-the-full-moon/ [Accessed 15 November 2015].

Arnett G. Global Peace Index 2014: Every Country Ranked. *The Guardian*. Website. 18 June 2014. Available from: http://www.theguardian.com/news/datablog/2014/jun/18/global-peace-index-2014-every-country-ranked [Accessed 12 March 2015].

Bailey JM. Book Review: Michael Jackson's Dangerous Liaisons. By Carl Toms. Padstow, Cornwall, TJ International, 2010. *Archives of Sexual Behavior*; 2011. DOI 10.1007/s10508-011-9842-1. Available from: http://faculty.wcas.northwestern.edu/JMichael-Bailey/articles/MJOCarroll-Review.pdf [Accessed 25 October, 2015].

Ball J. The Minnesota Starvation Experiment. *BBC World Service*. Website. 20 January 2014. Available from: http://www.bbc.co.uk/news/magazine-25782294 [Accessed 20 August 2015].

Bartholomew K, Kwong MJ, Hart SD. Attachment. In: Livesley WJ. (ed.) *Handbook of Personality Disorders: Theory, Research and Treatment.* New York: The Guilford Press; 2001. pp. 196–230.

BBC News. US Gunman James Holmes 'Legally Sane' At Time of Shooting. *BBC News US & Canada.* Website. 29 May 2015. Available from: http://www.bbc.com/news/world-us-canada-32936495 [Accessed 30 May 2015 and 2 June 2015].

Becker J. *The Chinese.* New York: Simon & Schuster; 2000.

Beers CW. *A Mind That Found Itself.* Pittsburgh and London: University of Pittsburgh Press; 1981.

Behuniak J. *Mencius on Becoming Human.* Albany: State University of New York Press; 2005.

Ben-Ami Bartal I, Decety J, Mason P. Empathy and Pro-Social Behavior in Rats. *Science.* 2011; 334(6061): pp. 1427–30.

Benko J. The Radical Humaneness of Norway's Halden Prison. *The New York Times Magazine.* Website. 26 March 2015. Available from: http://www.nytimes.com/2015/03/29/magazine/the-radical-humaneness-of-norways-halden-prison.html?_r=0 [Accessed 28 March 2015].

Bentham J. Selections from Bentham's Principles of Morals and Legislation. In: Bentham J, Mill JS. Ed. and Trans. by Troyer J. *The Classical Utilitarians.* Indianapolis / Cambridge: Hackett Publishing Company, Inc.; 2003. pp. 1–91.

Bering J. *Perv: The Sexual Deviant in All of Us.* New York: Scientific American / Farrar, Straus and Giroux; 2013.

Best J. Age of Consent Should Be Lowered to 15, Argues Leading Health Expert. *Mirror Online.* Website. 17 November 2013. Available from: http://www.mirror.co.uk/news/uk-news/lower-age-consent-15-argues-2801227 [Accessed 17 March 2015].

Binelli M. Inside America's Toughest Federal Prison. *The New York Times Magazine.* Website. 26 March 2015. Available from: http://www.nytimes.com/2015/03/29/magazine/inside-americas-toughest-federal-prison.html?_r=0 [Accessed 28 March 2015].

Black DW, Gunter T, Allen J, Blum N, Arndt S, Wenman G, Sieleni B. Borderline Personality Disorder in Male and Female Offenders Newly Committed to Prison. *Comprehensive Psychiatry*. 2007; 48(5): pp. 400–5.

Blakeway M. *The Logic of Self-Destruction: The Algorithm of Human Rationality*. York: Meyer LeBoeuf; 2014.

Blanchard R. Fraternal Birth Order and the Maternal Immune Hypothesis of Male Homosexuality. *Hormones and Behaviour*. 2001; 40(2): pp. 105–14.

Blanchard R, Kolla NJ, Cantor JM, Klassen PE, Dickey R, Kuban ME, Blak T. IQ, Handedness, and Pedophilia in Adult Male Patients Stratified by Referral Source. *Sexual Abuse: A Journal of Research and Treatment*. 2007; 19(3): pp. 285–309.

Blashfield RK, Reynolds SM, Stennett B. The Death of Histrionic Personality Disorder. In: Widiger TA. (ed.) *The Oxford Handbook of Personality Disorders*. New York: Oxford University Press; 2012. pp. 603–27.

Burton R. *The Anatomy of Melancholy*. New York: New York Review of Books; 2001.

Cantor JM, Klassen PE, Dickey R, Christensen BK, Kuban ME, Blak T, Williams NS, Blanchard R. Handedness in Pedophilia and Hebephilia. *Archives of Sexual Behavior*. 2005; 34(4): pp. 447–59.

Cantor JM, Kuban ME, Blak T, Klassen PE, Dickey R, Blanchard R. Physical Height in Pedophilic and Hebephilic Sexual Offenders. *Sexual Abuse: A Journal of Research and Treatment*. 2007; 19(4): pp. 395–407.

Castillo H. *Personality Disorder: Temperament or Trauma? An Account of an Emancipatory Research Study Carried Out by Service Users Diagnosed with Personality Disorder*. London and Philadelphia: Jessica Kingsley Publishers; 2003.

Chalmers DJ. Facing up to the Problem of Consciousness. In: Shear J. (ed.) *Explaining Consciousness, the Hard Problem*. Cambridge, MA: MIT Press; 1995. pp. 9–31.

Chalmers DJ. *The Conscious Mind: In Search of a Fundamental Theory*. Oxford: Oxford University Press; 1996.

Chalmers DJ. *Philosophy of Mind: Classical and Contemporary Readings*. New York: Oxford University Press; 2002.

Confucius. *The Analects*. Trans. by Waley A. London, New York, Toronto: Everyman's Library; 2001.

Corning WC, Balaban M. *The Mind: Biological Approaches to its Function*. New York: John Wiley & Sons Inc.; 1968.

The Council of States Governments, Justice Center. *Improving Outcomes for People with Mental Illnesses Involved with New York City's*

Criminal Court and Correction Systems. New York: Council of State Governments, Justice Center; 2012. Available from: http://csgjustice-center.org/wp-content/uploads/2013/05/CTBNYC-Court-Jail_7-cc.pdf [Accessed 26 November 2014].

Daly M, Wilson M. *Homicide.* New Brunswick, NJ: Transaction Publishers; 1988.

Daly M, Wilson M. Evolutionary Psychology of Male Violence. In: Archer J. (ed.) *Male Violence.* London and New York: Routledge; 1994. pp. 253–88.

Darwin C. On the Origin of the Species by Means of Natural Selection. In: Wilson EO. (ed.) *From So Simple a Beginning: Darwin's Four Great Books.* New York: WW. Norton & Company; 2005.

Darwin C. The Descent of Man, and Selection in Relation to Sex. In: Wilson EO. (ed.) *From So Simple a Beginning: Darwin's Four Great Books.* New York: WW. Norton & Company; 2005.

Darwin C. The Expression of Emotions in Man and Animals. In: Wilson EO. (ed.) *From So Simple a Beginning: Darwin's Four Great Books.* New York: WW. Norton & Company; 2005.

Davis C. Under the Bridge: The Crime of Living without a Home in Los Angeles. *The Intercept.* Website. 25 July 2015. Available from: https://firstlook.org/theintercept/2015/07/25/criminalizing-homelessness-in-los-angeles/ [Accessed 28 July, 2015].

Dawkins R. *The Extended Phenotype.* Oxford: Oxford University Press; 1982.

Dawkins R. *The Selfish Gene.* 30th anniversary ed. Oxford: Oxford University Press; 2006.

de Fruyt F, de Clercq B. Childhood Antecedents of Personality Disorders. In: Widiger TA. (ed.) *The Oxford Handbook of Personality Disorders.* New York: Oxford University Press; 2012. pp. 166–85.

de Waal F. *Chimpanzee Politics: Power and Sex among Apes.* Revised Edition 2000. Kindle Edition. Baltimore and London: John Hopkins University Press; 2007.

Dennett DC. *Brainstorms: Philosophical Essays on Mind and Psychology.* Montgomery, VT: Bradford Books, Publishers; 1978.

Dennett DC. *Elbow Room: The Varieties of Free Will Worth Wanting.* Cambridge, MA: The MIT Press; 1984.

Dennett DC. Quining Qualia. In: Marcel AJ, Bisiach E. (eds.) *Consciousness and Contemporary Science.* Oxford: Oxford University Press; 1988. pp. 42–77.

Dennett DC. *Darwin's Dangerous Idea: Evolution and the Meanings of Life*. New York: Simon & Schuster; 1995.

Dennett DC. Facing Backwards on the Problem of Consciousness. In: Shear J. (ed.) *Explaining Consciousness, the Hard Problem*. Cambridge, MA: MIT Press; 1995. pp. 33–6.

Dennett DC. Reflections on Free Will: A Review. *Sam Harris.* Weblog. 2014. Available from: http://www.samharris.org/blog/item/reflections-on-free-will [Accessed 27 January 2014].

Descartes R. *Discourse on Method*. Trans. by Clarke DM. London: Penguin Classics; 2000.

Dominguez RA. Treatment of Obsessive-Compulsive Disorder in Adults. In: Rush AJ. (ed.) *Mood and Anxiety Disorders*. Philadelphia: Williams & Wilkins; 1998. pp. 250–72.

Einstein A. *Relativity: The Special and General Theory. 100th Anniversary Edition*. Princeton: Princeton University Press; 2015.

Eissler K. Malingering. In: Wilbur GB, Muensterberger W. (eds.) *Psychoanalysis and Culture*. New York: International Universities Press; 1951. pp. 218–53.

Fazel S, Danesh J. Serious Mental Disorder in 23,000 Prisoners: A Systematic Review of 62 Surveys. *The Lancet.* 2002; 359(9306): pp. 545–50. doi:10.1016/S0140-6736(02)07740-1 [Accessed 18 June 2015].

Fonagy P, Luyten P. Psychodynamic Models of Personality Disorders. In: Widiger TA. (ed.) *The Oxford Handbook of Personality Disorders*. New York: Oxford University Press; 2012. pp. 345–71.

Ford M. America's Largest Mental Hospital Is a Jail. *The Atlantic.* Website. 8 June 2015. Available from: http://www.theatlantic.com/politics/archive/2015/06/americas-largest-mental-hospital-is-a-jail/395012/ [Accessed 12 June 2015].

Foucault M. *History of Madness*. Trans. by Murphy J, Khalfa J. London and New York: Routledge; 2006.

Freud S. *The Interpretation of Dreams*. 3rd ed. Trans. by Brill AA. New York: The Macmillan Company; 1913.

Freud S. *Three Contributions to the Theory of Sex*. 2nd ed. Trans. by Brill AA. Intro. by Putnam J.J. Ebook. New York and Washington: Nervous and Mental Disease Publishing Company; 1920. Available from: http://www.gutenberg.org/files/14969/14969-h/14969-h.htm

Futuyma DJ, Risch SJ. Sexual Orientation, Sociobiology, and Evolution. *Journal of Homosexuality.* 1984; 9(2–3): pp. 157–68.

Glynn I. *An Anatomy of Thought: The Origin and Machinery of the Mind*. Oxford: Oxford University Press; 1999.

Goldberg EM, Morrison SL. Schizophrenia and Social Class. *The British Journal of Psychiatry.* 1963; 109(463): pp. 785–802.

Greenwald G. *With Liberty and Justice for Some: How the Law is Used to Destroy Equality and Protect the Powerful.* Kindle Edition. New York: Metropolitan Books, Henry Holt & Co; 2011.

Gribbin J. The Thoughts of Stephen Hawking. *New Scientist*, No. 1621. 14 July 1988. p. 64.

Guillain G. *J.-M. Charcot, 1825–1893, His Life—His Work.* Ed. and trans. by Bailey P. London: Pitman Medical Publishing; 1959.

Gumert MD. Payment For Sex in a Macaque Mating Market. *Animal Behaviour.* 2007; 74: pp. 1655–67.

Hacking I. *The Social Construction of What?* Cambridge, MA and London: Harvard University Press; 1999.

Hamilton WD. The Genetical Evolution of Social Behaviour. I. *Journal of Theoretical Biology.* 1964; 7(1): pp. 1–16.

Hare RD. *Without Conscience: The Disturbing World of the Psychopaths among Us.* New York: Guilford Press; 1999.

Harris S. *The End of Faith: Religion, Terror and the Future of Reason.* New York: WW. Norton; 2004.

Harris S. *Free Will.* Kindle Edition. New York: Free Press; 2012.

Hegel GWF. Philosophy of Mind. Trans. by Wallace W. *Blackmask Online.* 2001. Available from: http://www.hegel.net/en/pdf/Hegel-Enc3.pdf [Accessed 17 September 2015].

Higgins ES, George MS. *Neuroscience of Clinical Psychiatry: The Pathophysiology of Behaviour and Mental Illness.* 2nd ed. Philadelphia: Lippincott, Williams & Wilkins; 2013.

Hirschfeld RMA, Vornik LA. Bipolar Disorder—Costs and Comorbidity. *The American Journal of Managed Care. 2005;* 11(suppl. 3). pp. S85–S90.

Hobbes T. *Leviathan.* London: Penguin Books; 1968.

Hooker E. The Adjustment of the Male Overt Homosexual. *Journal of Projective Techniques.* 1957; 21: pp. 18–31.

Horder J. *Excusing Crime.* Oxford: Oxford University Press; 2004.

Hume D. *A Treatise of Human Nature.* London: Penguin Books; 1969.

Hunter R, Macalpine I. *Three Hundred Years of Psychiatry: 1535–1860. A History Presented in Selected English Texts.* London: Oxford University Press; 1963.

Ingraham C. Why We Spend Billions to Keep Half a Million Unconvicted People Behind Bars. *The Washington Post.* Website. 11 June 2015. Available from: http://www.washingtonpost.com/news/wonkblog/wp/2015/

06/11/why-we-spend-billions-to-keep-half-a-million-unconvicted-people-behind-bars/ [Accessed 15 June 2015].

James DJ, Glaze LE. *Mental Health Problems of Prison and Jail Inmates.* Bureau of Justice Statistics Special Report. Washington, DC: U.S. Department of Justice; 2006. Available from: http://www.bjs.gov/content/pub/pdf/mhppji.pdf [Accessed 15 March 2015].

Jokela M, Batty GD, Vahtera J, Elovainio M, Kivimäki M. Socioeconomic Inequalities in Common Mental Disorders and Psychotherapy Treatment in the UK between 1991 and 2009. *The British Journal of Psychiatry.* 2013: 202(2): pp. 115–20.

Kane R. *Free Will and Values.* Albany: State University of New York Press; 1985.

Kierkegaard S. *Works of Love.* Trans. and eds. by Hong HV, Hong EH. Princeton NJ: Princeton University Press; 1998.

The Kinsey Institute. Frequently Asked Sexuality Questions to The Kinsey Institute. *The Kinsey Institute.* Website. 2015. Available from: http://www.kinseyinstitute.org/resources/FAQ.html#Age [Accessed 4 November 2015].

Koestler A. *The Sleepwalkers: A History of Man's Changing Vision of the Universe.* London: Pelican; 1968.

Kremer W. The Evolutionary Puzzle of Homosexuality. *BBC World Service.* Website. 18 February 2014. Available from: http://www.bbc.com/news/magazine-26089486 [Accessed 10 March, 2015].

Laing RD. *The Divided Self. An Existential Study in Sanity and Madness.* Intro. by David A. London: Penguin Books; 2010.

Lamperti J. *Does Capital Punishment Deter Murder? A Brief Look At the Evidence.* Hanover, NH: Dartmouth College; date unspecified. Available from: https://www.dartmouth.edu/~chance/teaching_aids/books_articles/JLpaper.pdf [Accessed 22 May 2015].

Lefkowitz MR, Fant MB. (eds.) *Women's Life in Greece and Rome: A Source Book in Translation.* 3rd ed. Baltimore: John Hopkins University Press; 2005.

Levi P. *The Drowned and the Saved.* London: Abacus; 1989.

Levin ED. The Rationale for Studying Transmitter Interactions to Understand the Neural Bases of Cognitive Function. In: Levin ED. (ed.) *Neurotransmitter Interactions and Cognitive Function.* Basel: Birkhäuser Verlag; 2006.

Levin ED, Rezvani AH. Nicotinic-Antipsychotic Drug Interactions and Cognitive Function. In: Levin ED. (ed.) *Neurotransmitter Interactions and Cognitive Function.* Basel: Birkhäuser Verlag; 2006.

Locke J. *An Essay Concerning Human Understanding.* Nidditch PH. (ed.). Oxford: Oxford University Press; 1975.

Lymburner JA, Roesch R. The Insanity Defense: Five Years of Research (1993–1997). *International Journal of Law and Psychiatry.* 1999; 22(3–4): pp. 213–40.

Mattia JI, Zimmerman M. Epidemiology. In: Livesley WJ. (ed.) *Handbook of Personality Disorders: Theory, Research and Treatment.* New York: The Guilford Press; 2001. pp. 107–23.

McDermott W, Zimmerman M. The Effect of Personality Disorders on Outcome of the Treatment of Depression. In: Rush AJ. (ed.) *Mood and Anxiety Disorders.* Philadelphia: Williams & Wilkins; 1998. pp. 321–38.

Merivale HC. *My Experiences in a Lunatic Asylum – by a Sane Patient.* Ebook. London: Chatto and Windus; 1879.

Mitchell AJ, Selmes T. Why Don't Patients Take Their Medicine? Reasons and Solutions in Psychiatry. *Advances in Psychiatric Treatment.* 2007; 13(5): pp. 336–46.

Morrison AP, Turkington D, Pyle M, Spencer H, Brabban A, Dunn G, Christodoulides T, Dudley R, Chapman N, Callcott P, Grace T, Lumley V, Drage L, Tully S, Irving K, Cummings A, Byrne R, Davies LM, Hutton P. Cognitive Therapy for People with Schizophrenia Spectrum Disorders Not Taking Antipsychotic Drugs: A Single-Blind Randomised Controlled Trial. *The Lancet.* 2014; 383(9926): pp. 1395–1403.

Mosendz P, Reuters. Robert Durst's History of Skipping Bail Comes Back to Haunt Him. *Newsweek.* Website. 23 March 2015. Available from: http://www.newsweek.com/robert-durst-jinx-denied-bail-316108 [Accessed 26 March 2015].

Nasar S. *A Beautiful Mind.* New York: Simon & Schuster; 1998.

Nisen M. The 10 Best Selling Prescription Drugs in the United States. *Business Insider.* Website. 28 June 2012. Available from: http://www.businessinsider.com/10-best-selling-blockbuster-drugs-2012-6?op=1 [Accessed 2 January 2014].

Nobel Prize. List of all Nobel Laureates in Physiology or Medicine. *Nobelprize.org.* Nobel Media AB 2014. Website. 2 March 2015. Available from: http://www.nobelprize.org/nobel_prizes/medicine/laureates/ [Accessed 3 March 2015].

Oades RD. Function and Dysfunction of Monoamine Interactions in Children and Adolescents with AD/HD. In: Levin ED. (ed.) *Neurotransmitter Interactions and Cognitive Function.* Basel: Birkhäuser Verlag; 2006.

O'Hara K, Scutt T. There is No Hard Problem of Consciousness. In: Shear

J. (ed.) *Explaining Consciousness, the Hard Problem*. Cambridge, MA: MIT Press; 1995. pp. 69–82.

Pincus AL, Hopwood CJ. A Contemporary Interpersonal Model of Personality Pathology and Personality Disorder. In: Widiger TA. (ed.) *The Oxford Handbook of Personality Disorders*. New York: Oxford University Press; 2012. pp. 372–98.

Pinker S. *The Blank State: The Modern Denial of Human Nature*. New York: Penguin; 2002

Pinker S. *The Language Instinct: How the Mind Creates Language*. New York: Harper Perennial Modern Classics; 2007.

Plato. The Timeaus. In: Jowett M. (ed. and trans.) *The Dialogues of Plato, in Five Volumes, Vol. III*. 3rd ed. London: Oxford University Press; 1892.

Plato. *The Republic*. In: Cooper JM, Hutchison DS. (eds.) *Plato: Complete Works*. Indianapolis / Cambridge: Hackett Publishing Company, Inc.; 1997.

Popper KR. *The Poverty of Historicism*. London: Routledge & Keagan Paul; 1957.

Popper KR. *Conjectures and Refutations: The Growth of Scientific Knowledge*. London: Routledge & Keagan Paul; 1963.

Popper KR. *The Open Universe: An Argument for Indeterminism*. London: Hutchinson & Co.; 1982.

Popper KR, Eccles JC. *The Self and Its Brain: An Argument for Interactionism*. Oxford: Routledge; 1984.

Porter R. *The Greatest Benefit to Mankind: A Medical History of Humanity from Antiquity to the Present*. London: Harper Collins; 1997.

Porter R. *Madness: A Brief History*. Oxford: Oxford University Press; 2002.

Powers M, Dalgleish T. *Cognition and Emotion: From Order to Disorder*. 2nd ed. Hove, Sussex: Psychology Press; 2008.

Rahman Q. The Association between the Fraternal Birth Order Effect in Male Homosexuality and Other Markers of Human Sexual Orientation. *Biology Letters*. 2005; 1(4): pp. 393–5.

Rahman Q, Hull MS. An Empirical Test of the Kin Selection Hypothesis for Male Homosexuality. *Archives of Sexual Behavior*. 2005; 34(4): pp. 461–67.

Ronningstam E. Narcissistic Personality Disorder: The Diagnostic Process. In: Widiger TA. (ed.) *The Oxford Handbook of Personality Disorders*. New York: Oxford University Press; 2012. pp. 527–48.

Rothenbuhler WC. Behaviour Genetics of Nest Cleaning in Honey Bees. IV. Responses of F1 and Backcross Generations to Disease-Killed Brood. *American Zoologist*. 1964; 4(2): pp. 111–23.

Rousseau J-J. *Confessions.* (Translator unknown). London, New York, Toronto: Everyman's Library; 1992.

Rousseau J-J. A Discourse on the Moral Effects of the Arts and Sciences. In: Ryan A. (ed.), Cole GDH. (trans.) *The Social Contract and the Discourses.* London, New York, Toronto: Everyman's Library; 1993. pp. 1–30.

Rousseau J-J. A Discourse on the Origin and Basis of Inequality amongst Men. In: Ryan A. (ed.), Cole GDH. (trans.) *The Social Contract and the Discourses.* London, New York, Toronto: Everyman's Library; 1993. pp. 31–126.

Rousseau J-J. The Social Contract or Principals of Political Right. In: Ryan A. (ed.), Cole GDH. (trans.) *The Social Contract and the Discourses.* London, New York, Toronto: Everyman's Library; 1993. pp. 181–98.

Russell B. *A History of Western Philosophy.* London: Allen & Unwin; 1961.

Ryle G. *The Concept of Mind.* London: Penguin (Peregrine Books); 1978.

Sade Marquis de. *Justine, or the Misfortunes of Virtue.* Trans. by Phillips J. Oxford: Oxford University Press, Oxford World Classics; 2012.

Sandfort T. *Boys on Their Contacts with Men: A Study of Sexually Expressed Friendships.* New York: Global Academic Publishers; 1987.

Saraceno B, Levav I, Kohn R. The Public Mental Health Significance of Research on Socio-Economic Factors in Schizophrenia and Major Depression. *World Psychiatry.* 2005; 4(3): pp. 181–5.

Sarter M, Bruno JP, Parikh V, Martinez V, Kosak R, Richards JB. Forebrain Dopaminergic-Cholinergic Interactions, Attentional Effort, Psychostimulant Addiction and Schizophrenia. In: Levin ED. (ed.) *Neurotransmitter Interactions and Cognitive Function.* Basel: Birkhäuser Verlag; 2006. pp. 65–86.

Scull A. A Convenient Place to Get Rid of Inconvenient People: The Victorian Lunatic Asylum. In: King AD. (ed.) *Buildings and Society: Essays on the Social Development of the Built Environment.* London, Routledge; 2005. pp. 19–31.

Schwirtz M. Rikers Island Struggles with a Surge in Violence and Mental Illness. *The New York Times.* Website. 18 March 2014. Available from: http://www.nytimes.com/2014/03/19/nyregion/rise-in-mental-illness-and-violence-at-vast-jail-on-rikers-island.html?hp&_r=0 [Accessed 12 November 2014].

Shephard B. *A War of Nerves; Soldiers and Psychiatrists, 1914–1994.* London: Jonathan Cape; 2000.

Szasz TS. *The Manufacture of Madness: A Comparative Study of the Inqui-*

sition and the Mental Health Movement. New York: Syracuse University Press; 1997.

Szasz TS. *The Myth of Mental Illness: Foundations of a Theory of Personal Conduct.* Ebook. New York: Harper Collins; 2011.

Torgersen S. Epidemiology. In: Widiger TA. (ed.) *The Oxford Handbook of Personality Disorders.* New York: Oxford University Press; 2012. pp. 186–205.

Torrey EF. *Out of the Shadows: Confronting America's Mental Illness Crisis.* New York: John Wiley & Sons; 1997.

Torrey EF, Kennard AD, Eslinger DF, Biasotti MC, Fuller DA. *Justifiable Homicides by Law Enforcement Officers: What is the Role of Mental Illness?* Arlington, VA: Treatment Advocacy Center and the National Sherrifs' Association; 2013. Available from: http://tacreports.org/storage/documents/2013-justifiable-homicides.pdf [Accessed 3 April 2015].

Trivers R. *Social Evolution.* Menlo Park CA: Benjamin Cummings; 1985.

United States Census Bureau. U.S. and World Population Clock. *United States Census Bureau.* Website. 2015. Available from: http://www.census.gov/popclock/ [Accessed 15 March 2015].

von Neumann J. The Mathematician. *Works of the Mind.* I(I). Chicago: University of Chicago Press; 1947. pp. 180–96.

Walmsley R. *World Pre-Trial/Remand Imprisonment List (Second Edition).* London: International Centre for Prison Studies; 2014. Available from: http://www.prisonstudies.org/sites/default/files/resources/downloads/world_pre-trial_imprisonment_list_2nd_edition_1.pdf [Accessed 16 June 2015].

Widiger TA, Samuel DB, Mullins-Sweatt S, Gore WL, Crego C. An Integration of Normal and Abnormal Personality Structure: The Five-Factor Model. In: Widiger TA. (ed.) *The Oxford Handbook of Personality Disorders.* New York: Oxford University Press; 2012. pp. 82–107.

Winerip M, Schwirtz M. Rikers: Where Mental Illness Meets Brutality in Jail. *The New York Times.* Website. 14 July 2014. Available from: http://www.nytimes.com/2014/07/14/nyregion/rikers-study-finds-prisoners-injured-by-employees.html?_r=1 [Accessed 12 November 2014].

Wittgenstein L. *Tractatus Logico-Philosophicus.* Trans. by Ogden CK. London: Routledge & Keegan Paul; 1922.

Wittgenstein L. *Philosophical Investigations.* Trans. by Anscombe GEM. Oxford: Basil Blackwell Ltd; 1953.

Wittgenstein L. *Lectures & Conversations on Aesthetics, Psychology and Religious Belief.* Oxford: Blackwell Publishing; 1966.

World Health Organization. *International Statistical Classification of*

Diseases and Related Health Problems, 10th Revision. Chapter V, Mental and Behavioural Disorders. World Health Organization. Online Standard Diagnostic Tool. 2015. Available from: http://apps.who.int/classifications/icd10/browse/2015/en

Zhisui L. *The Private Life of Chairman Mao.* New York: Random House, Inc.; 1994.

ABOUT THE AUTHOR

Matthew Blakeway studied philosophy, mathematics and formal logic before pursuing a career in investment banking. He structured and modified financial derivatives and complex financing mechanisms in an industry where the reverse engineering of competitors' systems is common practice. After twenty years spent analysing and manipulating abstract conceptual frameworks, he began to develop a theory that humans are abstract mechanisms and that we, too, can be reverse engineered. *The Logic of Madness* is the culmination of that journey of discovery.

ACKNOWLEDGEMENTS

Anastasia Said provided copy-editing and editorial assistance. Becky Ferriera and Julie Jackson also provided editorial input. Kristen Harrington of the Curved House coordinated production. Emma King designed the front cover, and Eric J. Henderson was the photographer.

Stephen Baines, Steve Matteo and my sister Clare provided substantial practical and logistical assistance throughout the writing and production of this book.

INDEX

By the same author

The Logic of Self-Destruction
The algorithm of human rationality

Why do knowingly act in ways that undermine our own wellbeing, like loving the wrong person or staying in an unfulfilling job? Why are ideologies so compelling? Why are we so convinced that our own, deeply held views are irrefutable? The Logic of Self-Destruction argues that our beliefs are at the heart of our problems, and that if we can see the human brain for what it really is – a robustly logical, computing device, we can finally understand how those beliefs are really formed.

Matthew Blakeway's jovial and engaging multidisciplinary argument applies a logician's rigour to genetics, linguistics, socio-biology and evolutionary psychology, to investigate the unique human ability to affect and suppress emotions. In showing how everything from the British stiff-upper-lip to abusive relationships, from the rise of fundamentalist regimes to the failure of economies, stem from this problem, he provides new tools for understanding our motivations and shaping our futures.

- In The Logic of Self-Destruction, Matthew Blakeway takes the reader on a fascinating journey through the logic of human behaviour. He uses a series of thought experiments based in everyday situations to reveal how we manipulate our emotions tactically – as individuals, social tribes and societies – and explores the consequences of this.

- He challenges the assumption that happiness is an innate, instinctive human emotion and demonstrates what mystical 'higher states of being' have in common with art appreciation.

- He investigates the suppression of emotional behaviour in groups to explain how humiliation on the parade ground turns a soldier into a killer, and how totalitarian regimes are perpetuated.

- He reveals why ideology is more powerful than scientific evidence, and explains why climate change denial and even genocide can be explained rationally.

Reviews of *The Logic of Self-Destruction*

"Via a series of thought experiments, Blakeway offers a fascinating journey through evolutionary theory, philosophy and psychology. While assuming that humans are robustly logical, he explains self-destructive actions and ideological beliefs. From an innovative analysis of the Holocaust to reflections on rising fundamentalism, his argument is convincing."

(Claire Fletcher-Flinn, Frontiers in Psychology)

"There's something rather fin de siècle about 2014, and nowhere more so than in philosophy books. Matthew Blakeway's The Logic of Self-destruction: The Algorithm of Human Rationality (Meyer LeBoeuf) is an ambitious survey."

(Martin Cohen, editor of The Philosopher, nominates his book of the year 2014, Times Higher Education)